Medicine & Society
In America

Medicine & Society
In America

Advisory Editor

Charles E. Rosenberg
Professor of History
University of Pennsylvania

Disease And Society
In Provincial Massachusetts

Collected Accounts,
1736-1939

*A*RNO *P*RESS & *T*HE *N*EW *Y*ORK *T*IMES
New York   1972

Reprint Edition 1972 by Arno Press Inc.

LC# 73-180563
ISBN 0-405-03948-4

Medicine and Society in America
ISBN for complete set: 0-405-03930-1
See last pages of this volume for titles.

Manufactured in the United States of America

CONTENTS

Caulfield, Ernest
A TRUE HISTORY OF THE TERRIBLE EPIDEMIC VULGARLY CALLED THE THROAT DISTEMPER WHICH OCCURRED IN HIS MAJESTY'S NEW ENGLAND COLONIES BETWEEN THE YEARS 1735 AND 1740

Dickinson, Jonathan
OBSERVATIONS ON THAT TERRIBLE DISEASE VULGARLY CALLED THE THROAT-DISTEMPER, WITH ADVICES AS TO THE METHOD OF CURE. In a Letter to a Friend

Douglass, William
THE PRACTICAL HISTORY OF A NEW EPIDEMICAL ERUPTIVE MILIARY FEVER, WITH AN ANGINA ULCUSCULOSA WHICH PREVAILED IN BOSTON NEW-ENGLAND IN THE YEARS 1735 AND 1736

Fitch, Jabez
AN ACCOUNT OF THE NUMBERS THAT HAVE DIED OF THE DISTEMPER IN THE THROAT, WITHIN THE PROVINCE OF NEW-HAMPSHIRE, WITH SOME REFLECTIONS THEREON, July 26, 1736

A TRUE HISTORY OF THE
TERRIBLE EPIDEMIC VULGARLY CALLED
THE THROAT DISTEMPER
WHICH OCCURRED IN
HIS MAJESTY'S NEW ENGLAND COLONIES
BETWEEN THE YEARS 1735 AND 1740

TO
GROVER F. POWERS

A TRUE HISTORY
of the
TERRIBLE EPIDEMIC

VULGARLY CALLED
THE THROAT DISTEMPER

WHICH OCCURRED IN
His Majesty's New England Colonies
BETWEEN THE YEARS 1735 AND 1740

By

ERNEST CAULFIELD, M.D.

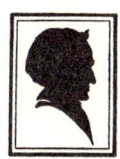

Published for the BEAUMONT MEDICAL CLUB
by the
Yale Journal of Biology & Medicine
New Haven, Connecticut
1939

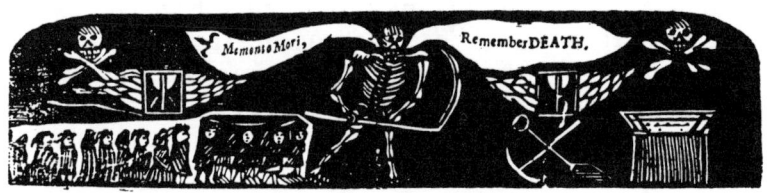

> Both Young and Old, O come behold
>   the Works which God hath wrought,
> The fearful Desolation, which
>   he on this Land hath brought.
> —Awakening Calls to Early Piety.

Almost as far back as written records go we find evidence that mankind has been afflicted by frequent recurrences of horrible epidemics. Periodically occurring without any apparent cause, each one has taken its toll of life and then departed as strangely as it came. They have halted social progress, determined the results of wars, and sometimes even threatened the existence of civilization itself. Nearly every age has witnessed some distressing disease in epidemic form. Leprosy and influenza were prevalent at the time of the Crusades and the Black Death of the Middle Ages is said to have destroyed one-fourth the population of the earth. The plague closed the theatres and retarded the full development of Elizabethan culture, and numerous other outbreaks followed down to the end of Stuart times. Smallpox and dysentery epidemics frequently occurred throughout the eighteenth century. Not so long ago, influenza spread rapidly around the world. We now fear the return of infantile paralysis. And so it goes.

It has long been known that there was an epidemic of some disease in Kingston, New Hampshire, in 1735, but it is not so well known that this was merely a small part of a greater epidemic which involved most of the inhabited regions of New England and caused great loss of life wherever it appeared. To that generation of Americans it was a new disease and to them its behaviour was as strange as it was mortal. In some of the towns nearly half of all the children died and at times it was feared that the disease would actually destroy the colonies. It drove the people to their churches to meditate and pray, and special fast days were proclaimed in Massachusetts and in Connecticut. *"How terrible hath GOD been in his Doings,"* they cried, "Numerous Families have been emptied. A great Number of the *Children are cut off from without, and the young Men from the Streets* . . . We may reasonably conclude that GOD is giving of us Warning to prepare for all Events."

The excitement that prevails at the time of epidemics is usually in proportion to the severity of the disease. As an example, we have only to remember the infantile paralysis epidemic in New England in 1931. At first it was regarded as an unavoidable nuisance, but in a very short time the reports became more alarming. In spite of all precautions it continued to spread nearer and nearer to home and soon we were very much concerned. Then appeared the screeching headlines, pictures of dying children in mechanical respirators, long lists of horrible and dangerous symptoms, and frantic appeals for donors of blood. In a few months all was quiet again and when the statistics were compiled it was found that among every two hundred thousand people about ten deaths had occurred. Let us now compare this with the "throat distemper" of eighteenth century New England. That epidemic continued for at least five years and among an equal number of people about five thousand deaths occurred. Except in a very few towns, however, one finds no evidence of any great confusion, and certainly there was not the loss of self-control that people usually exhibit during great epidemics of this kind. Perhaps this apparent outward calm did not truly reflect the inward feelings of the people, but there is good reason to believe that it did, for with implicit faith in God they did not question the meaning or justice of their misfortunes. That they were submissive and composed may be one reason why most historians have overlooked this terrible disaster, although it was a major epidemic in the annals of this country and caused more deaths than any pre-Revolutionary war. But it seems that the emotions were only temporarily suppressed, for immediately following these five years of sickness and death, indeed, so close in time that a causal connection might be suspected, there occurred a period of intense excitement,— that great psychological and religious upheaval better known as "The Great Awakening."

Outside of Boston and its environs, New England in 1735 consisted of numerous small isolated towns, each with from two hundred to five thousand inhabitants. Products of the garden, field, and forest were brought to the larger towns, especially those along the coast, but except for an occasional fair, where produce, sheep, and cattle were bartered and except for help in the protection against Indian raids, each of the smaller frontier towns was self-supporting and independent of its neighbor. Although in the very early days most of the homes were grouped around the church and the central common, by 1735, particularly where the Indians were no longer feared, many of the homes were far from the center of the town and often widely separated from each other. Each family had its own supply of water, milk, and other foods and could live in comfortable seclusion even through the long cold winters when snowbound for many weeks. Therefore, it seems somewhat strange that an epidemic of a contagious disease could gain much headway because the means were at hand for an almost complete isolation had the most elementary precautions been enforced. But there was more to life than mere existence on a farm, and there were many complicating factors that might explain the spread of a disease.

To appreciate one complicating factor, one must consider the prevailing theories of contagion, best illustrated by the treatment of smallpox which was very common at that time. When a case occurred in Boston, for example, the patient was sent to either Spectacle or Rainsford Island where the province maintained pesthouses for the isolation and treatment of contagious cases. At one time, a house in the sparsely settled west end of the town was converted into a hospital and, while patients were there for treatment, a guard was thrown around the house and a red flag was hoisted to warn visitors of the danger. Ships coming from infected ports were stopped in the harbor, thoroughly inspected, and the crew and passengers were frequently detained until all danger of infection had subsided. Most of the provinces had stringent laws to prevent the spread of smallpox and other contagious diseases. In Rhode Island, the penalty for violation of the sanitary code was death "without benefit of clergy." It was also known that a person was generally immune following an attack of smallpox and was therefore less liable to spread the disease. Nurses and attendants had to prove that they had been previously infected and a pock-marked slave had an increased value at the market. The intense controversy that followed the introduction of inoculation in 1721 was not only about the immunizing value of inoculation, but also about the danger of an inoculated case to other people. No one doubted that smallpox could be contracted by direct exposure to another case. Contagion, however, was not so readily apparent when there were epidemics of those diseases that we now know are spread by healthy carriers and when all the facts could not be readily explained the whole contagion theory was hastily abandoned. This accounts for the fact that the "throat distemper" was treated as a very strange disease and as one that did not spread by contact. The rapid progress of the epidemic can be partly attributed to this error in judgment, but the error itself was the result of other circumstances.

The interpretation of medical facts concerned the physician most of all and in this period all manner of men called themselves physicians. First, there was the quack. He existed in eighteenth century New England just as he has existed in all other times and places. Perched upon a platform he extolled the virtues of his secret drug, while a two-piece band squeaked forth some simple tunes and a well-trained dog leaped through a paper hoop. But he cleverly managed to perform his cures in towns where there were no epidemics, so he can be neither praised nor blamed for anything that happened. Opposed to the quack was the physician who made an honest effort to improve both himself and his profession. With the welfare of his patients at heart he studied his cases, listened with respect to the opinions and advice of others, and then fearlessly expressed his own conclusions. During this epidemic there was one such man in particular who stood above the others,—William Douglass, a Boston physician, wrote a detailed account of his experiences and in doing so made a valuable contribution to the existing medical literature of the world. The great majority of physicians, however, were of the country doctor type,—kindly, honest, diligent, respected. As there were no medical schools in this country, most of them acquired their skill in blistering, bleeding, and prescribing from preceptors, whose knowledge consisted chiefly of an intricate arrangement of the folk-lore of the times. The professional reputation of the doctor was measured by his ability to memorize a lot of ineffectual remedies or to control the dosage of a violent puke or purge, but he was sincere in his efforts and even if he stumbled while he went groping for the truth, he must be greatly admired for his undaunted courage in the face of many difficult tasks. When confronted with this epidemic of an apparently new disease he carried on against overwhelming odds, but partly because of inadequate training and partly because of misinterpretation of the facts, it was the country doctor who first decided that the disease was not contagious and who was, therefore, responsible in a large measure for the spread of the disease.

The best educated man in the New England town was the minister, who, spending many hours with the sick and dying, soon acquired the medical knowledge of the day and often applied it quite successfully. In towns where there were no physicians, the ministers tended bodies as well as souls, and during the "throat distemper" epidemic we find such men as Parson Smith of Falmouth, Hugh Adams of Durham, John Tucke of the Isles of Shoals, Nathaniel Williams of Boston, and Thomas Toucey of Newtown (Conn.) playing the double rôle. In fact, it was Jonathan Dickinson, a minister-physician, who wrote one of the best medical treatises on the "throat distemper." But even when the minister did not practice medicine, he was the acknowledged leader in the interpretation of extraordinary events, and when the people sought the explanation of anything unusual he seldom hesitated to expound upon the first causes of all things. To be sure, Cotton Mather was dead and a bit of liberalism had somewhat softened the fire-and-brimstone theories of an earlier day, but the people still gave a religious interpretation to every event of their daily lives and still considered each adversity as a just punishment for sin. During the many days of fast and prayer they humbly reflected upon the "especial Sins wch God is angry wth ye Land & with us for." One can find very little evidence of bitterness or complaint. As a natural result of a century of Puritanism there was no conflict between their theology and their science. When this epidemic began, science and theology agreed. Science failed, and when it could not adequately explain all the facts, the people turned to theology for assistance in their distress. But it was this readiness to adopt a theological explanation for the epidemic which was chiefly responsible for the hasty abandonment of a scientific one.

The ministers and physicians were factors in the spread of this disease in another way. They were in physical contact with the sick and carried the infection on their clothes and hands to their own families, at least, and probably all around the town. Doubtless some of them were healthy carriers. One of the very noticeable characteristics of the "throat distemper" epidemic is the frequent occurrence of many deaths in the families of the ministers and physicians.

Because this epidemic spread chiefly among the children, some aspects of their lives need to be considered. Since the middle of the seventeenth century, the law had decreed that towns with more than fifty householders must provide for childhood education and by 1735, public schools were firmly established throughout New England. Schoolhouses were one-room buildings and during the winter months the children huddled about the open fire. Those whose parents contributed a share of wood were given the choice seats, but if the spread of an epidemic was in direct proportion to exposure, then the pupils who sat off in chilly corners by themselves were in somewhat less danger of contracting the disease. On Sundays, trailing their elders along the road or mounted with them upon a horse, the children went to church. They accompanied their parents to the church door, but a strict ritual demanded that within, the children must sit together at the rear or in the gallery. A tithing man watched over them and attempted to prevent their restlessness and disorders during the two- or three-hour sermons. The unruly youngsters ran noisily up and down the stairs and in and out of church; occasionally they "sported and played, and by indecent Gestures and Wry Faces, caused laughter and misbehaviour in the Beholders, and thereby greatly disturbed the Congregation." After church there was again the temptation to play. The boys threw stones at the meeting-house windows and "profaned the Sabbath" in many other ways. The evidence indicates that the children, at least, did not wear long faces, but frequently played together, particularly on Sundays, when they undoubtedly contracted many of their contagious diseases.

Funeral ceremonies of colonial New England have been frequently described. We need not be concerned about the order of procession, the gifts of mourning rings and gloves, or the tolling of the bells, but reading between the lines we find some means by which a disease could spread. The funeral of a child was an occasion when all the playmates and younger relatives of the deceased were brought together. Children acted as bearers in the long march to the grave; they came into close contact with the corpse and no attempt was made to separate the healthy mourners from the other infected children of the afflicted family.

Thus a child's life on a solitary farm was not so isolated as one might at first suppose. The conditions were almost perfect for a contagious disease to spread, and when the "throat distemper" epidemic appeared in one of these old New England towns, its beginning was as explosive as it was malignant.

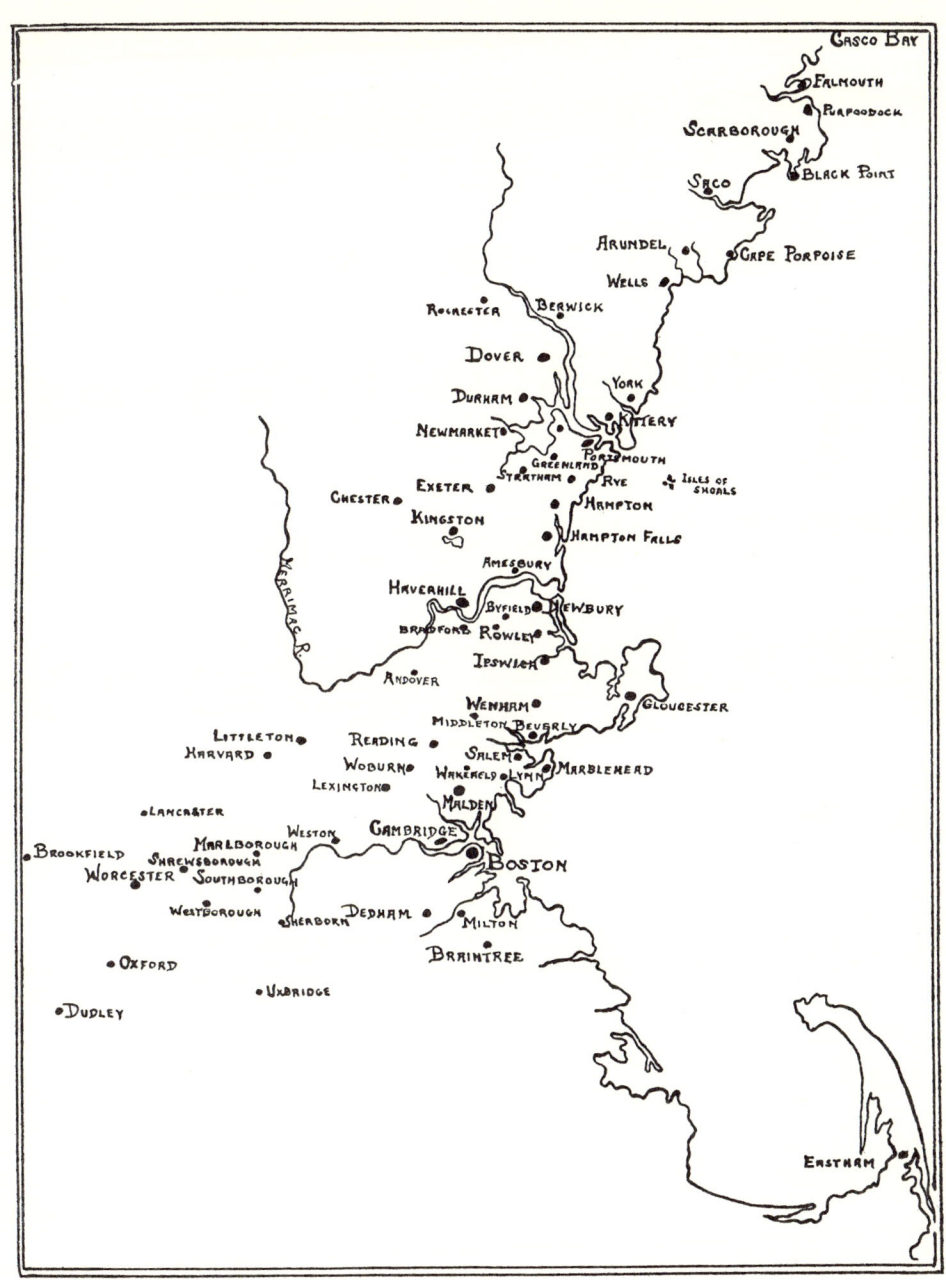

I

KINGSTON, NEW HAMPSHIRE

> It makes me weep in sorrows deep,
>   to hear the dying moans,
> Which Death has made, in these our Days,
>   among our little Ones.
> —A Lamentation.

Fifteen miles north of the Merrimac River and about the same distance from the coast is a little fresh water lake which has been known for a long time as "The Great Pond." Nearby lies the town of Kingston, famous in that part of New Hampshire as the ancestral home of Daniel Webster and the adopted home of Josiah Bartlett, physician, Governor of New Hampshire, and, according to tradition, the first to sign the Declaration of Independence. Even without any very unusual scenery Kingston, nevertheless, has the charm of a peaceful, sleepy, quaint New England town with its few old colonial homesteads set back from a road that encircles "Kingston Plaine," the shaded village green.[1] Across the road, eastward from the green, is the old burying ground with its scattered groups of brown moss-covered stones. Some are overturned, others partly crumbled or buried in the earth, but their distinctive shapes, grimly smiling cherubs, and ornamental borders mark them as relics of early colonial days. Although most of them are difficult to read, an occasional inscription identifies these stones as marking the graves of children who died during an epidemic when Kingston was a thriving town on the western frontier of New England civilization.

About the middle of the seventeenth century when the English began to extend their frontiers inland, they found the Indians inhabiting the country surrounding "The Great Pond," for it was good hunting ground and the land was more fertile than was the sandy soil nearer to the coast. The early settlers met with prolonged and stubborn resistance from the natives, but by 1694 the country had become sufficiently populated to warrant a charter for a township which was to be called "Kingstowne" in honor of William of Orange, then King of England. After many rigorous winters and frequent raids by hostile tribes, the town began to thrive and by

---

[1] George H. Moses: *The Road-Encircled Plain: A Sketch of Kingston*. *Granite Monthly*, 1894, xvii, 351.

the time of George the Second about four or five hundred people had selected this region for their homes.

Among the eighty-one families of Kingston in 1725, the names of Bean, Clifford, Ladd, Prescot, Samborn, and Webster are found most frequently; some of them, direct descendants of the earliest settlers, had lived there for many years. The boundaries of the town were not well defined and included the greater part of the present Sandown, Danville, and East Kingston. By this time, the people had learned to face their hardships with resolute determination and had overcome many of the difficulties of earlier frontier life. They had no particular trade, but like other New Hampshire people raised their own livestock, barley, corn, and wheat; cut their own timber and brought it on ox-carts to the mill. The average family possessed a horse, four cows, and four or five hogs. Salting down the pork in preparation for the long cold winter was as important as gathering the harvest in the fall, and so, to Bostonians, these people soon became known as "great pork eaters" which, after all, was not a very distinctive characteristic, for it was common to the inhabitants of most of the other inland New England towns. At that time, Kingston was almost self-sufficient and an occasional "pedalar" or visiting relative was the only contact with the outside world. There were no wars or famines, the scene of Indian raids had shifted to the west and north, and, except for a perennial argument with their southern neighbors about the Massachusetts boundary-line, the people were as content and happy as the Puritan conscience would allow.

To this small group of sturdy, upright, farming people, the Rev. Ward Clark was called to be the minister when the church was organized in 1725.[2] Since his graduation from Harvard College (M.A., 1723), he had taught a grammar school in Exeter, his native town, a few miles to the north, but he was still only twenty-two when he undertook his new assignment and proudly entered in his book the names of his parishioners, headed by the Esquires, Captains, Ensigns, and Lieutenants. A leader in fostering community pride, he himself planted most of the elms that later shaded the village green. This kindly young man, able to interpret liberally a rigid Calvinistic doctrine, was devoted to his work and his efforts were soon rewarded with the admiration and respect of an apprecia-

---

[2] Rev. J. H. Mellish: *Historical Address on the 150th Anniversary of the Kingston Congr. Church.* 1876, 12.

tive congregation. Pleased with £80 a year, a home, and the prospects of a permanent settlement, he married Mary Frost of Kittery in 1727. During the first ten years of his ministry a new and larger meeting-house was built, for a hundred and thirty new members had joined the church and the population of the town had almost doubled, many of the new settlers coming from neighboring towns in northeastern Massachusetts. During the same period there were about eighty marriages and four hundred baptisms; Clark's salary was increased many times and he was granted liberal tracts of land. There had been a small epidemic of some childhood disease during the autumn and winter of 1730-31, but now the usual good health again prevailed and the minister and people of Kingston, with many of their earnest hopes fulfilled, looked forward to a tranquil and satisfying future.

Spring seems always late in coming to New England, but it was later than usual when it reached New Hampshire in 1735. It was said that the weather was uncomfortably wet and cold and that easterly winds prevailed. As the tradition goes,[3] in April of that year, one of the hogs that belonged to a Mr. Clough was "taken sick with a complaint in its throat and died. Mr. Clough skinned the hog and opened it. Soon after, he was taken with a complaint in his throat, and died suddenly." But this is probably mere tradition, because there is no record of the death of Mr. Clough in 1735. However, on May 20, 1735, Parker Morgan, the son of John Morgan, died after a few days' sickness. About a week later, in a house four miles away, Nathaniel, John, and Elizabeth, the three children of Jeremiah Webster, died within three days. There was something unusual about the deaths of these four children, each with the same short illness. Some blamed the unseasonable weather; others knew it was a warning from an angry God; all agreed that it was very strange. The events of June are effectively told in the stark realism of the parish records:[4]

June y^e	5	Deborah Child of Josiah Batchelor Died
	7	Dorothy Daughter of Jacob Gilman Died
	17	Samuel Lock Lost a Daughter
	18	Ebenezer Sleeper Lost a son. Both died with a Quinsey
	19	Samuel Emons Eldest Daughter Died
	21	Died David son of Joseph Greely

---

[3] J. Farmer and J. B. Moore: *Collections, Topographical, Historical and Biographical relating principally to New Hampshire.* 1822, i, 143.

[4] *Kingston Church Records: New Hampshire Geneal. Record,* ii, 43; iii, 37.

23	Samuel Emons lost another
23	The Same Day Ebenezer Sleeper Lost another
25	Andrew Webster Lost his Child
25	Joseph Bean lost one of His Children
27	Died another of Joseph Beans Children
28	Died Margaret Eldest Daughter of Joseph Bean
30	Samuel Emons Lost another Child

By the end of June the people were very much alarmed, for only once, in 1730, had the deaths for a whole year exceeded the deaths for this one month. This strange "Plague in the Throat" was not like any disease with which they were familiar. They knew that whooping-cough and measles could spread among children, but never had any such mortality accompanied a childhood epidemic. They could understand smallpox epidemics because that disease spread by contact, but this one attacked here and there "not according to the effects of contagion or qualities of the soil" and so was beyond their understanding. Soon it was certain that "God hath been provoked to visit this People with sore and grievous Calamities," so the young minister quickly summoned his afflicted people to fast and pray together.

Meanwhile, the disease had invaded many other homes and July only brought increased sorrows.

July ye 1^{rst}	Died Nathaniel youngest son of m^r Jos^e Greely
4	Died Daniel son of John Huntoon
8	Died Isaac Son of Isaac Godfrey
10	Died William Another son of Isaac Godfrey
11	Died Nathaniel the Other son of Isaac Godfrey
11	Died Gideon son of John Yonng
14	Died a Daughter of Benjamin French
16	Rachel Died Daughter of Richard Tandy
17	Died Caleb Webster Brother of Jeremiah Webster
19	Died William ye Eldest son of William Smith
22	Died Mary Youngest Child of John Huntoon
26	John Webster Lost a Child
27	Died ye Wife of ye Revd Mr Ward Clark and her Infant
28	Died Moses ye son of Deacon Elkins
28	Ralph Plazdel Lost a Child
29	William Smith Lost an other Child
31	Jacob Flanders Lost a Child
31	Died Henery Youngest son of Deacon Elkins

There are no detailed accounts of those hot, distressing, summer days in Kingston. So far as known, nothing was done to prevent the spread of the disease. If the first few cases had occurred in neighboring homes, perhaps the people would have suspected that the disease was spread by contact, but the first cases were four miles apart and the disease kept reappearing in widely separated sections of the town without any apparent reason, so it was decided that this "Strange unusual Distemper" was the "Fruit of strange Sins" and contagion was not thought to be a factor.[5] Up to this time the remedies of Dr. Simeon Brown and Dr. Green had failed in every case. Bleeding, blistering, and purging had invariably hastened death and the long-tried and favorite remedies seemed to have suddenly lost their power. Only the "Tenders and Watchers" could soften the distress. In spite of the "Many Days of Fasting and Prayer that were observed in the Beginning of this fatal Calamity," the disease raged on through August:

August y^e	1	Obediah Elkins Lost a Child
	6	Obediah Elkins Ther other Child
	7	William Buzzel Lost a Child
	9	John Clifford Lost a Child
	10	Eliz: Daughter of Samuel Colcord Died
	11	Saml Bean Lost a Child
	11	Dr Brown lost a Child an Onely Daughter
	11	Joseph Elkins Lost His Eldest Daughter
	12	Died Ruth Daughter of Simon French
	13	Serg^t William Buzzel Lost another Child
	14	Daniel Bean Lost a young Son
	14	Joseph Elkins Lost Another of their Children
	15	Joseph Elkins Lost Another of their Children
	15	Jacob Flanders Lost another Child
	16	Died Thomas Son of Jedidiah Philbrick
	19	John Clifford Lost another son 14 years old
	19	Joshua Prescut Lost a young daughter
	21	Joshua Prescut Lost another
	22	Joseph Elkins Lost his other Child
	23	Died John Clark Son of ye Revd Mr Clark
	23	Died a Son of Jonathan Samborn
	26	Died Benjamin Clark Son of ye Revd Mr Clark
	27	Robert Stockman Lost a Child
	27	John Clifford Lost another
	31	Samuel Bean Lost another a Daughter
	31	Benjamin Sweat Lost His Eldest Child

---

[5] Jabez Fitch: *An Account of the Numbers that have died . . . within the Province of New Hampshire.* Boston, 1736, 13.

In September, at last, it seemed that the prayers were answered. There were only six deaths compared with twenty-six in August, but in October there was another increase to fifteen, twelve of whom were children. With six deaths in November and eight more in December, the total stood one hundred and two for the year, whereas since records had been kept the yearly average had been less than ten.[6] No detailed descriptions of the disease have been found, but written into the church records at the close of 1735 is this simple entry:

This Mortality was By a Kanker Quinsey or Peripn[eumony], which mostly Seized upon young People and has Proved Exceeding mortal in Several other Towns y^t It is supposed there never was y^e like Before in this Country.

Tradition says that many died within twelve hours and that others, while sitting up at play, would fall and expire with their playthings in their hands.[7]

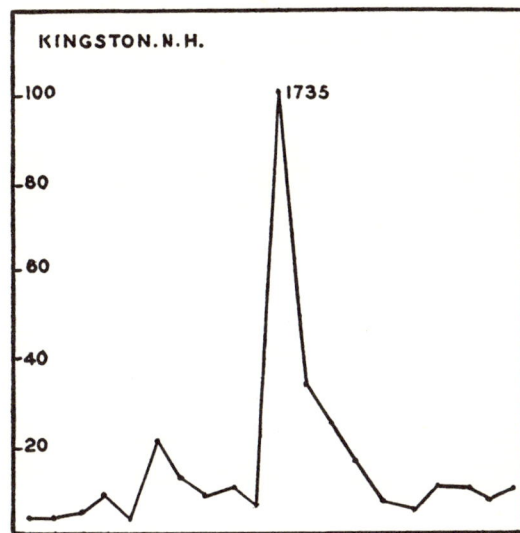

Kingston, N. H., deaths, 1725-1744. Compiled from records in the *Coll. New Hamp. Hist. Soc.*, 1837, v, 250.

The epidemic continued through 1736, when there were thirty-four deaths including that of "Eliz. Clark y^e only Daughter of Revd Mr Clark" on August 29th. With twenty-four deaths in 1737 and sixteen in 1738, it was not until after 1739 that the death-rate resumed average proportions. The epidemic had spent itself, but it had visited most of the families in the town and left many of them childless. Within a year, one family lost all four, another lost four out of six, and six families lost three each.[8] Of the first forty who were taken sick, not a single

---

[6] Ora Pearson: *Mortality in Kingston from 1725 to 1832. Coll. N. Hamp. Hist. Soc.* 1837, v, 250.

[7] Farmer and Moore: *loc. cit.*

[8] Jabez Fitch: *An Account* . . . etc. p. 5.

one recovered[9] and more than a third of all the children in the town had died.[10] Yet of all the affliction and distress in Kingston, no one suffered more than the minister, Ward Clark. He had fought adversity with an unfaltering sense of duty, but had lost his wife and four children, and all his efforts had ended in disaster. He could endure no more. Broken in health, he returned to his native Exeter, where he hoped to regain his strength under the care of Dr. Deane, a relative and practising physician. He drew up his will in which he remembered the poor and his "Beloved people of Kingston" and soon after, on May 6, 1737, at the age of thirty-four, he died of a "wasting consumption," probably some lingering complication of the disease.

II

NEW HAMPSHIRE

This strange Disease doth mostly seize
those that are young and tender,
And 'tis so smart, it strikes the Heart,
and makes 'em to surrender.
—A Lamentation.

In 1735, most of the inhabitants of the Province of New Hampshire lived in the territory that lies between the Merrimac and Piscataqua Rivers and that extends inland for about twenty miles. A few of the fifteen or twenty towns were already about a century old, for very soon after the Pilgrims had landed at Plymouth there were settlements along the Piscataqua at the present sites of Dover and Portsmouth, and Exeter and Hampton were founded a little later by settlers from Massachusetts Bay. The other towns were relatively new, having sprung up during the early eighteenth century, chiefly as separated parishes of the older towns. It is a pleasant country, yet unspoiled by modern trade, and to one with any regard for the charms of the colonial period there are few more delightful places than old Portsmouth or the country-side along the "Kings Great Road" to Exeter.

When the news of the Kingston epidemic spread to the surrounding towns it is probable that many outsiders avoided Kingston,

---

[9] William Douglass: *The Practical History of a new Epidemical . . . Fever.* Boston 1736, 1.

[10] Mellish: *loc. cit.* says "nearly all of the young children."

for man generally fears an epidemic of disease, but after it was decided that the disease was not contagious it is also probable that many others went to Kingston to assist their unfortunate relatives and friends. We now know that some diseases are transmitted by healthy people as well as by direct contact with the sick, so with such a virulent and widespread focus as Kingston it might be expected that the disease would soon appear in the neighboring towns.

Today, Hampton Falls is fifteen miles east of Kingston, but in 1735, although the intervening country was already settled, they were adjoining towns. The present town of Kensington, which was established in 1737, was then the western part of Hampton Falls and East Kingston was separated from Kingston in 1738. The list of petitioners for the separation of East Kingston[11] includes the names of many families that lost children when the epidemic began, so that the disease had to spread only to a neighboring house in order to involve a family that attended church at Hampton Falls. In this way an entirely separate town could become infected. This was the probable course of events, because an epidemic started in Hampton Falls in June, a few weeks after the disease broke out in Kingston.

The Hampton Falls epidemic reached its peak during the winter months and during December alone there were fifty deaths. This town suffered more than any other in New Hampshire, and within about a year two hundred and ten had died, of whom two hundred were under twenty years of age. One family lost seven children, two families lost six, two lost five, six lost four, and about fourteen families lost three apiece.[12] The disease was still present in 1739 when Joseph Batchelder lost twelve or thirteen children,—it was not known which,—for "Mrs. Batchelder afterwards was unable to decide whether she had twelve or thirteen children." It was also said that only two houses where there were children escaped the epidemic.[13]

---

[11] *New Hampshire Town Papers.* Edited by I. W. Hammond. Concord, 1884, xii, 334.

[12] Jabez Fitch: *An Account* . . . pp. 2-6. Unless otherwise indicated, New Hampshire statistics have been taken from this source.

[13] Warren Brown: *Hist. of Hampton Falls*, 301. According to the *Boston News-Letter*, however, (Mar. 28-April 5, 1739), Joseph Batchelder lost six children.

Hampton Falls, then a town of about two hundred houses and twelve hundred people, had been separated from the old town of Hampton in 1726. It had grown more rapidly and become more of a trade center than Kingston, since it was on the main road that led through New Hampshire southward to Salisbury and Newbury in the province of Massachusetts Bay. A fair, which attracted people from neighboring towns, was held at the Falls two or three times a year and travellers on their way to Maine often stopped at the inn and mingled with the people of the town, so when Hampton Falls became a second focus there was an opportunity for the disease to spread even beyond the borders of the province.

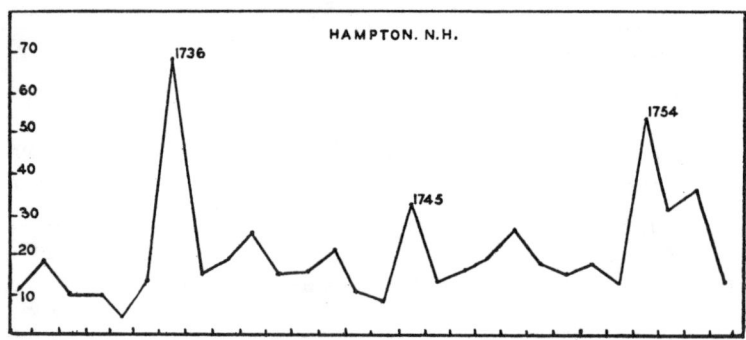

Hampton, N. H., deaths, 1730-1757. Recurrences of "Throat distemper." Compiled from records in Belknap: *Hist. New Hamp.*, iii, 178; *New Engl. Hist. & Geneal. Reg.*, 1904, lviii, 29.

In contrast to Hampton Falls, the first parish of Hampton, which was north of Taylor River and contained the same number of people, had only fifty-five deaths from the distemper within the first year and about eighty for the years 1735-37. The Hampton church records contain a brief first-hand account of the disease:

July y[e] 26, 1735 on Saterday my Brother Samuels daughter abigil was taken ill with a mortal distemper: the tuesday following which was the 28 day of July his only son Sam[ll] was taken with the same awfull illness they continued till Saterday and both died: august y[e] 2nd abigil early in y[e] morning and Sam[ll] early that evening they were lovely in their life and in their death they were not devided: they were decently buried in one grave on monday aug 4th and on tuesday morning his daughter Elisabeth died after about three days after she was taken with the same distemper the distemper dreadfully siezed their throat in an awfull manner.[14]

---

[14] *New Engl. Hist. & Geneal. Reg.*, 1904, lviii, 31.

THE "THROAT DISTEMPER" OF 1735-1740

By August, 1735, the disease had spread to Exeter, six miles to the north, and another conflagration burned with all its devastating fury. Within a year there were one hundred and twenty-seven deaths, all but nine among children under fifteen years of age. Exeter was an older and much larger town than Kingston and, although it appears that the epidemic was not as extensive in proportion to the population, the disease was just as mortal in the particular homes where it occurred. With utter disrespect for the remedies of those days it even crossed the threshold of the home of Dr. Deane, the chief physician of the town:[15]

    Deborah Deane died Sept. 6 1735
    Sarah   "   "   "   15   "
    Abigail   "   "   "   18   "
    Mary   "   "   "   19   "

Stratham, Greenland, and Newmarket, small towns near Exeter, each had about twenty deaths.[16]

In September the disease broke out in Durham, and within a few months another hundred deaths was added to the rapidly growing list. Now up to this time the cause of the epidemic had remained obscure and even the doctors who were supposed to know all about such things were forced to admit that they were helpless. According to a contemporary poem:

> The Doctor's Art, can find no part,
>   nor Cure for this Distemper;
> By Physick long, nor Cordials strong,
>   they cannot find the Center.
>
> It is unknown to any one
>   and all the Doctors skill,
> To cure this Plague, or to engage
>   to cure it at their will.
>
> They're in the dark, in every part,
>   and cannot find it out,
> From whence it strikes, and where it lights
>   they cannot point it out.
>
> If we should call the Doctors all
>   and let them all engage,
> We cannot find in any kind
>   that they can cure this Plague.

---

[15] Ibid: 1883, xxxvii, 289.

[16] For the 1742 recurrences of the epidemic in Greenland and Stratham, see: *New Engl. Hist. & Geneal. Reg.*, xxix, 38; xxx, 427; xxxii, 48.

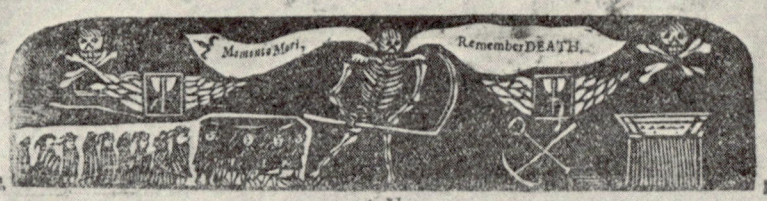

AN ELEGY

Upon the much lamented DEATHS of two desireable Brothers, the two eldest Sons of

Capt. Joshua and Mrs. Comfort Weeks,

Of Greenland;

Who departed this Life in *February* 1735,6. the youngest whose Name was *Ichabod*, died the 3d Day, in the 22d Year of his Age, and the eldest whose Name was *Joshua*, deceased the 10th Day, in the 24th Year of his Age, leaving his honoured Parents and a desireable Widow with other near Relations in mournful Tears. Let us all that are yet spared, improve this and the many other Warnings that we have had in the Year past, remembering the Command of CHRIST is, *Be ye also ready.*

Respected Friends, my heart is griev'd
That of your Sons you are Bereav'd!
But pray don't be Disconsolate,
 Altho' your Loss is very great;
But with GOD's Dealings be content,
Knowing your Children were but lent.
GOD Righteous is in calling home,
Those Comforts which from him did come.
GOD often has unto us shown,
That He has Power to take his own,
When young and small or when up-grown
 'Tis Comfort, your's did live so long,
To show they did to GOD belong.
I trust GOD did their Souls remove,
For to enjoy their Saviour's love.
Then if your loss, to them be gain,
I pray take care not to complain.
But thankful he, that GOD has given
Such hopes, your Sons are gone to Heaven.
What greater Comfort can you have,
Than hopes that GOD their Souls did save.
Surely this may your Comfort be,
That they from failings were so free,
And that by GOD they were inclin'd,
 their own immortal Souls to mind.
These many years I have them known,
Good Inclinations they have shown.
This plainly show'd what was their Care,
Their daily using Secret Prayer,
And practising such secretly,
I trust was true sincerity.
I pray it may your Comfort be,
What in your Sons you did often see;
That they behav'd themselves so well,
That to their Praise we may it tell.
They were to Parents Dutiful,
And each was thoughtful of his Soul.
They shew'd themselves obedient,
'Till Sickness was upon them sent,
And when they on their Death-bed lay,
They did most readily obey.
They were two kind and loving Brothers,
More than is common among others.
What grieved one, grieved the other's Heart,
'Twas but one Week Death did them part,
And then they both were laid in Ground,
I trust both Souls have Mercy found.
Now pray let this your Comfort be,
Such Hope, they're from all troubles free.
Let this also some Comfort grant,
That they Renew'd their Covenant,
And with their Duty did comply,
And also walked orderly.
Under your loss pray Imitate
God's Saints who have had Losses great.

David tho' after GOD's own Heart,
Of Losses sure he had his Part,
For one he griev'd before 'twas dead,
So that he would not eat his Bread:
But when he found Death was GOD's Will,
He did submit with Silence still:
But David after mourned more,
The Aggravations being sore,
Having no Hopes of him at all,
Who did in his Rebellion fall.
Such Cause to mourn you cannot have,
Because you have Hopes beyond the Grave.
Consider too whom GOD did call
A perfect Man, and yet lost all,
And in his Loss did bless the Lord,
As is recorded in his Word.
Pray imitate such blessed Saints,
Who never dar'd to make Complaints,
What's done is by a Holy GOD,
I pray submit unto the Rod,
And cleave to him who does correct,
As well becomes GOD's own Elect.
My Friend, who now art lonesome left,
Being of your bosom friend bereft,
I pray don't be discouraged,
Your GOD still lives, tho' Husband dead:
Cleave close to him who surely can,
You comfort more than any Man:
Take Comfort in GOD's Promises
Made unto Widows that are in.
Will GOD to you a Husband be
Who can you from all Troubles free
What can a greater Comfort be?
Are not GOD's Promises now more
To you than e'er they were before?
Then now go on and serve the Lord,
And trust to you fulfil his Word,
Tho' you have lost a tender Friend,
GOD can you comfort to the End;
Therefore from GOD don't turn aside,
And you will have your Wants supply'd.
Brothers and Sisters that remain,
Pray by this Loss, your Souls may gain.
Your Brothers Counsels left behind,
Do not forget, but always mind;
And of your Souls in time take care.
And daily seek
That he for Heav
Your Saviour striv
More than on Earth
You see that Riches
Those that enjoy them,
What Profit can in them
After the Body's in the Ground.

Now let us set by Earth more light,
And seek Heaven with all our Might;
And not to set our Hearts upon,
Earth's Comforts, which may soon be gone.
You see what GOD hath lately done,
Improve it well, pray every one,
And now GOD's Will is done, 'tis fit,
That you with Silence all submit,
And not to mourn with great Excess,
Lest that GOD's Laws you should transgress;
And yet we must such Notice take,
That we may right Improvement make,
Remembering 'tis a Warning given,
To wean from Earth and fit for Heaven.
Don't GOD to us now loudly say,
Make ready for your dying Day.
You see that Life uncertain is,
Dangerous for to delay it is,
The Call to all now seems to me,
See that you also ready be.
Such Calls then don't let us despise,
But for our Souls learn to be wise;
And prepare for Eternity,
Knowing we all must surely die.
GOD does sometimes our Branches take,
That we more fruitful he may make.
Then let us drive more Fruit to bear,
When we by GOD so pruned are.
GOD sometimes brings Afflictions
Upon his Daughters and his Sons,
To show them the Uncertainty,
Of all such Comforts as must die;
That they on Him might set their Love,
And on those Things that are above;
Which only will true Comfort yield,
When other Comforts all have fail'd,
When Streams of earthly Comforts dry,
Let us unto the Fountain fly.
Where we may have a full Supply,
Of Grace to help aright to bear,
When we under Afflictions are.
To you that do in *Greenland* live,
GOD does this awful Warning give
To others all in ev'ry Town,
By Youths and Children soon cut down
GOD does unto us often call,
For to forsake our Evils all,
And speedily without Delay
Prepare for the great Judgment-Day
For all a strict Account must give,
How here upon the Earth they live,
And have Reward accordingly,
Of Happiness or Misery.

F I N I S.

(Courtesy of the New Hampshire Historical Society.)

There was one man in Durham, however, who could explain this mysterious disease. Hugh Adams, "Clerk, the Gospel Minister and Pastor of the Church at Durham" was a graduate of Harvard College (1697) and had combined the practice of medicine with his preaching in many towns before he contracted with the Durham parish for his "ministerial labours." Soon afterwards the currency became inflated and the Durham people, unlike the people in other towns, made no effort to please their minister with regular increases in salary, for the simple reason, as it later became apparent, that they didn't enjoy his preaching and they sometimes even went so far as to withhold his salary altogether. Bitterly complaining about this "sacrilegious fraud" and at the same time proving that he was gifted with extraordinary powers, Adams finally petitioned the Governor and General Court. He stated that on one occasion when his arguments about his salary had not produced results, he had prayed that it would not rain, and, very probably to his own surprise, there was not a drop of rain for three months! Then a few remaining friends protested that they were innocent victims and that their own crops were nearly destroyed, so Adams obligingly reconsidered and declared a private fast when for a full day he "abstained three meals from *eating, drinking* and *smoaking* anything." Immediately, there were "repeated plentiful and warm rains, as recovered the languishing corn, grass and fruits of the trees, unto a considerable harvest thereof; so as was then remarkable ..." Furthermore, according to the petition, good ministers were appreciated in Massachusetts and the laws of that province demanded that they should be promptly and adequately paid, but there were no such laws in New Hampshire. No wonder, Adams said, that an epidemic was raging in New Hampshire while Massachusetts was relatively free.[17] The poem continues:

> Let's search the Cause, 'tis breach of Laws,
>   that punishes for Sin,
> That brings down Plagues in every Age,
>   as it has ever been.
>
> Ungrateful Sins have ever been
>   most odious in GOD's Sight,
> Then let's repent with one consent,
>   and pray both Day and Night.[18]

---

[17] Belknap: *Hist. of New Hamp.*, 111: 263.
[18] *A Lamentation.*

Beyond Durham, the road to the north leads into Dover, where the sickness began in October, 1735, and caused eighty-eight deaths before the following July. In March, 1736, the *Boston News Letter* reported: "Last Saturday four Children lay dead in one House at Dover, who died of this mortal Sickness." At another time four other children of one family were buried in the same grave and there were two or more deaths in many families throughout that winter and spring. The epidemic even reached the small remote settlement at Rochester, where Nathaniel Ham and his brother, the first two children born in the town, died of "throat distemper" and were buried in the same grave.[19]

Chester was a small town of about four hundred people out in the "Chestnut Country" west of Kingston, and during 1735-36, although there were only twenty deaths, considerable attention was given to the Chester phase of the epidemic. It was supposed that a contagious disease would spread rapidly in all directions. From Kingston, this disease had spread to Hampton Falls on the east by June, to Exeter on the north by August, but it was not until October that it reached Chester on the west. That puzzled everyone and together with the strange behaviour of the disease in other towns the evidence now seemed convincing that this disease was not contagious. If the people had considered other facts they would have found some evidence that it was, because the epidemic could be seen spreading to the north at a definite rate per day. Starting from Kingston in June, it reached Exeter in August, then ten miles north to Durham in September, and then ten miles further north to Dover in October. But they repeatedly overlooked such facts and emphasized exceptions. Throughout the subsequent history of the epidemic the contagion theory occasionally reappears, but every time that it does some contrary evidence arises to overthrow it.

Portsmouth, with about three or four thousand people, was the cultural, financial, and governmental center of New Hampshire. Most of the provincial trade with foreign countries passed through this town and there was frequent contact with the people in neighboring towns, so it is surprising, therefore, to find that Portsmouth escaped the epidemic until nearly all the other towns had become infected. In a sermon preached during the winter of 1735-36,[20] it

---

[19] McDuffie: *Hist. of Rochester,* 44.
[20] Jabez Fitch: *Two Sermons on the . . . Fatal Distemper.* Boston, 1736, 10.

was said that the mortal sickness, though present, did not prevail to the same extent as in other towns; and it was not until January that a Portsmouth epidemic was first mentioned in the contemporary press. On February 9, the *Boston Evening Post* reported:

> We are informed, that 7 Children died at Portsmouth the last Week, and that 3 children of Mr. Thomas Bickford of that Place, and which were all that he had, were buried together on Wednesday last.

Subsequently, very conflicting accounts appeared. In March, the *Boston News-Letter* mentioned that the epidemic had been "pretty favourable at Portsmouth hitherto," but later that month it was as "mortal as in any of the neighboring Towns" and seventy had died within a short time. By April the epidemic had "considerably abated," but by July the number of deaths had reached one hundred. There was a pest-house in Portsmouth at this time and in 1736 the provincial government allowed an increased appropriation for its maintenance.[21] Here is indirect evidence that Portsmouth physicians may have treated the distemper as a contagious disease and, if it is supposed that the first few cases were immediately isolated, the small number of deaths during 1735 can possibly be explained. But it does not seem that a single pest-house could have been effective for very long because it would surely have been overtaxed with the seventy fatal cases during the late winter, so it is probable that the isolation treatment in Portsmouth was ineffectual. Certainly it cannot explain the fact that, in proportion to the population, Portsmouth had fewer deaths than any other New Hampshire town.

Jabez Fitch (1672-1746), the minister at the North Church in Portsmouth, wrote a valuable account of the New Hampshire epidemic. Born in Norwich, Connecticut, the fourth son of the Rev. James Fitch, he attended Harvard College (1694) and was a tutor and a fellow there. A few years at Ipswich was followed by "a pious and useful ministry of more than twenty years continuance" in Portsmouth, where he died of a "nervous fever" in 1746. Fitch had been impressed by the epidemic and went to most of the neighboring towns to gather mortality statistics. Although

---

[21] *New Hampshire Provincial Papers.* 1722-1737, iv, 723. Edited by N. Bouton.

published as a theological work, *An Account of the Numbers that have died of the Distemper in the Throat, Within the Province of New Hampshire* is a commendable piece of scientific research and is of great value to epidemiology, for it not only gives the total numbers that died in the various towns but the deaths are grouped according to age. In eighteenth century medical publications one usually has to allow for errors in interpretation, but these statistics are reliable because there could have been very little chance for error in recording a child's age at the time of death. Naturally, Fitch was interested in a theological interpretation of his figures and when he found that the disease vented its fury chiefly upon the children he attributed it to "the woful Effects of Original Sin." We need not be concerned with the religious aspect of this work, but we will have further occasion to refer to the statistics.

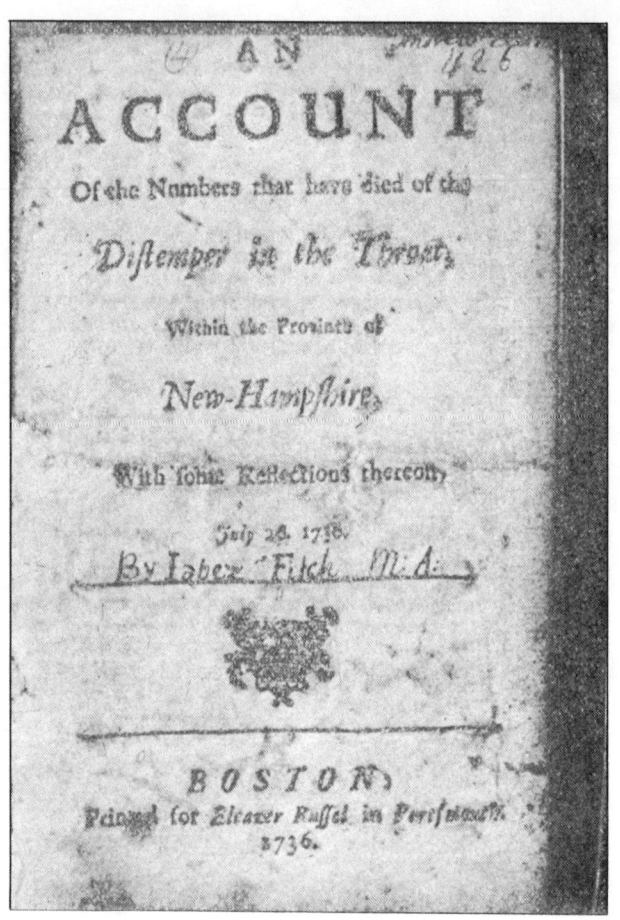

(Courtesy of the Boston Athenæum.)

Towns	Under 10	10 to 20	Over 20	Total
Portsmouth	81	15	3	99
Dover	77	8	3	88
Hampton	37	8	10	55
Hampton Falls	160	40	10	210
Exeter	105	18	4	127
Newcastle	11			11
Gosport	34	2	1	37
Rye	34	10		44
Greenland	13	2	3	18
Newington	16	5		21
Newmarket	20	1	1	22
Stratham	18			18
Kingston	96	15	2	113
Durham	79	15	6	100
Chester	21			21
	802(81.5%)	139(14.1%)	43(4.3%)	984

Deaths in New Hampshire, modified from Belknap's compilation of Fitch's statistics.[22] As there were very few deaths in June, 1735 (13 in Kingston and a few more in Hampton Falls), and as the "Account" probably went to press early in July, 1736, I have taken these figures to be the approximate number of deaths for the first year of the epidemic (July 1, 1735-July 1, 1736). In addition to Fitch's figures, the newspapers[23] reported that "several" died at Derry and Nottingham.

The "Account of the Numbers . . ." was published July 26, 1736, and many, especially local, historians have accepted the figures as complete. But when Fitch wrote, the epidemic was not over, indeed, one month later the *Boston News-Letter*[24] reported: "The Distemper is yet very bad at Portsmouth and many dye of it. It is attended with a violent fever." The records of various churches, while they do not mention the exact cause of death, indicate that the distemper was still prevalent after Fitch's work was printed. For instance, in Rye, just south of Portsmouth, Abner, Jacob, Mary, and Tryfenny Lock all died in July-August 1736.[25] At least fifty died in the course of a year in this parish of three hundred souls.

---
[22] J. Belknap: *Hist. of New Hamp.*, ii, 94.
[23] *Boston Evening Post*, Feb. 16, 1736; *New York Gazette*, March 6-15, 1735/6. Deaths in New Hampshire estimated at 600 up to Jan. 30, 1736. Statistics for various towns given.
[24] August 26-Sept. 2, 1736.
[25] *New Hamp. Geneal. Record.* July, 1903, i, 43. Multiple deaths in the Berry, Doust, Goss, and Marden families also.

There are records of the epidemic at Newcastle, an island at the mouth of the Piscataqua River, and even among a small,

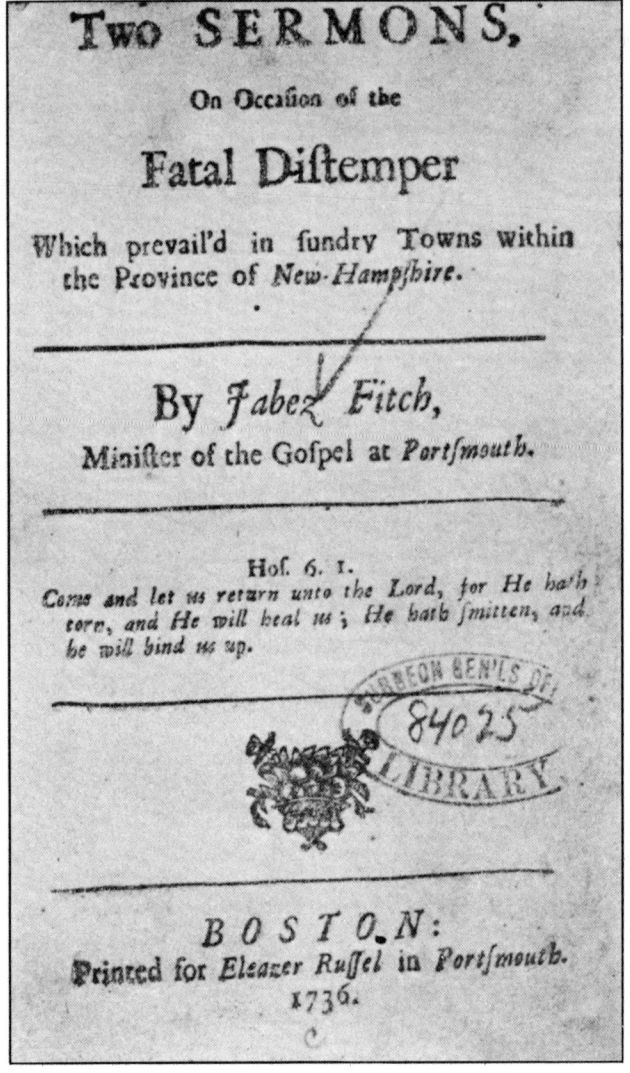

(Courtesy of the Surgeon General's Library.)

isolated colony of fishermen on the wind-swept Isles of Shoals, eight miles at sea, thirty-six children died of the distemper during the winter and spring of 1735-36.

III

MAINE

> To Newbury O go and see
> To Hampton and Kingston
> To York likewise and Kittery
> Behold what God hath done.
> —Awakening Calls to Early Piety.

Maine was a part of Massachusetts Bay Province at that time, but for convenience the Maine towns are treated as a separate group. Most of them were small fishing towns at occasional harbors between the Piscataqua River and Casco Bay and their total population was less than nine thousand.

The epidemic began in Kittery in June, 1735, which was very soon after it began in Kingston, but this could not have been a direct spread across the Piscataqua River from the vicinity of Portsmouth for the epidemic had not yet reached that region. The appearance of the disease in Kittery, as in Chester and other places, was difficult to explain and such unusual events made Jabez Fitch decide:

> The Progress of the late Distemper has been very strange in its passing from one Town to another, after a considerable space of Time, and in its long remaining in one Part of a Town, before it has pass'd into other parts, and in its returning where it seem'd to be quite gone, and the Fears of it were blown over; on these Accounts the Act of Providence is the more visible in sending it, and we are led to look beyond natural Causes to the Hand of God, to whom we are chiefly concern'd to apply our selves for the Removal of this awful Calamity.

History does not say that "Vice, Pride, Envy, Malice & Evil-Speakings" were any more common in Kittery than elsewhere, so modern science attempts to explain this mystery in some other way. There could easily have been some direct connection between Kittery and Kingston. Ward Clark's wife (Mary Frost) came from Kittery, his brother had lived in Kittery and there were probably other families with equally close connections. During the exciting times in June, some friend or relative may have gone to Kingston, contracted the disease in a mild form and then returned. Although in apparent good health, that person could still harbor the disease. Or, some person in Kingston may have gone to Kittery and become sick a few days after his arrival. Later we shall find a specific instance in which the disease was carried to Boston in this manner.

Again, our knowledge of the healthy carrier can account for the apparent mystery without any reference to Kingston, for the disease may have been carried to Kittery from Hampton Falls where an epidemic also began in June. A traveller on his way from Boston to Maine may have become infected as he stopped to rest and gossip at the Hampton Falls Inn, and a day or two later, as the people of Kittery gathered around him for news of the distemper, the very germ that caused it might have been disseminated with every word. It is no wonder that the progress of the epidemic seemed so strange.

The news that Kittery was involved spread up the coast and each town prepared to defend itself. Parson Smith of Falmouth wrote in his journal:

> Oct. 31, 1735. We had a Fast ... on account of the sickness which broke out at Kingston, N. H., and which is got as far as Cape Porpoise, and carries off a great many children and young persons and alarms the whole country.[26]

That same month other fasts were held at York[27] and Berwick[28] to prevent the spread of the disease, but the fasts were answered "by terrible things in Righteousness" and the settlements at Spruce Creek,[29] York, and Wells[30] soon became involved. From the reports it cannot be determined when the epidemic appeared in the various towns, but there are records of it at Arundel (Kennebunk),[31] Cape Porpoise, Saco, Black Point (Prout's Neck), Scarborough,[32] Purpoodock (Cape Elizabeth and South Portland),[33] Falmouth

---

[26] *Journal of the Rev. Thomas Smith*, Portland, 1894. Contains brief references to the epidemic in various Maine towns.

[27] C. E. Banks: *Hist. of York*, Boston, 1931, i, 354, 367. *Boston News-Letter*, March 11-18, 1736. The Rev. Mr. Moody is supposed to have written an account of the epidemic in York. (Mentioned in John Brown's *Relation*. 1737.)

[28] J. C. Scates: *Records of the First Church of Berwick*. N. E. Hist. & Geneal. Reg., 1928, lxxxii, 97.

[29] *Boston News-Letter*, March 11-18, 1736.

[30] E. E. Bourne: *Hist. of Wells & Kennebunk*, p. 351.

[31] *Boston News-Letter*, Jan. 22-27, 1737. New Eng. Hist. & Geneal. Reg., 1889, liii, 123. George March of Kennebunkport "lost seven children in one week." Seven children of Joseph Averell and of Jane McLellan, his wife, died in 1735. *The Averell Family*, p. 170.

[32] *Boston News-Letter*, Jan. 22-27, 1737. "Not one has lived that has had it of late"—Smith.

[33] 26 deaths before May 1737,—Smith. The Rev. Benjamin Allen lost five children within a week.

(Portland),[34] Casco Bay,[35] Presumscot Falls, North Yarmouth,[36] and Pemaquid.[37]

The epidemic continued for many months. June 16, 1736, was a day of fasting and prayer at the First Church in Falmouth on account of "the terrible distemper that has been and is still prevailing in the land." Practically all of the parishioners were present and it was an unusually solemn affair. Parson Smith, physician as well as minister, made frequent notes in his journal about those days of sickness and mentions that the epidemic was still present in 1737 and 1738. No first-hand descriptions of the Maine disease have been found. At Scarborough there were times when the mortality approached one hundred per cent. It has been estimated that there were five hundred deaths in Maine,[38] which is probably not an exaggerated estimate in view of the more than one hundred and twenty-five deaths in Kittery alone.[39]

IV

BOSTON

> But not to go so far,
> the daily 'counts we hear,
> Are 'nough to fill a thinking Soul
> with trembling Dread and Fear.
>
> —Earnest Expostulation.

Late in the summer of 1735, the disease that had "as yet no proper Name assign'd to it" invaded the northern part of Massa-

---

[34] 40 deaths before May 1737,—Smith.

[35] *Boston News-Letter*, March 11-18, 1736.

[36] Including Freeport and Harpswell. Lydia Tuttle d. Dec. 7, 1736—"The first by throat distemper." Multiple deaths in the Anderson, Brown, Burnell, Fogg, Ingersol, Larrabee, Seabury, Weare, and Winslow families. *Ms. Record of Deaths*, in Maine Hist. Soc.; *Old Times in North Yarmouth*. Jan. 1884, p. 1105. According to Smith's *Journal* there were 75 deaths before May, 1737. I have been unable to locate: "*A Poem on the Death of Martha Chandler of North Yarmouth*," a broadside, Boston, 1737. She died in August, 1737, probably from the "throat distemper."

[37] William Douglass—*Practical History* ... p. 13. *Virginia Gazette*, Apr. 28-May 5, 1738.

[38] Williamson: *Hist. of the State of Maine*. 1832, ii, 186.

[39] Fitch: *An Account* ... p. 6. *Boston Evening Post*, Nov. 24, 1735.—"the Distemper still prevails at Kittery, &c, and a Child of Col. Pepperil's about 3 Years old, died of it last Friday."

chusetts. By this time a large part of New Hampshire was infected and, as there were no quarantine restrictions, the disease could be carried into Massachusetts by countless travellers going to many different towns. As a matter of fact, the epidemic appeared in various Massachusetts towns at different times and its exact course cannot be traced in geographical or chronological sequence. Moreover, the descriptions of the Massachusetts cases differ in some important particulars from the case descriptions in New Hampshire so that, on the whole, the Massachusetts epidemic seems very complicated and for a correct interpretation of the contemporary records it is first necessary to establish the diagnosis. There are clear and accurate accounts of the disease as it appeared in Boston, therefore it is more profitable to describe the situation there and defer the histories of the intervening towns.

There had been rumors in Boston about the strange and mortal "Eastern Distemper," but there was no alarm while it remained so far away. Late in September, however, when the epidemic had actually crossed the Merrimac River, it seemed that Boston would inevitably become infected and the selectmen became very much disturbed. Boston had just recovered from a serious smallpox epidemic which occurred five years before, trade was good and the general health was better than it had been for many years, so the selectmen were determined that if possible they would avoid another siege of sickness at this time. Consequently, they invited the leading physicians to their council meeting on October 1, for it was earnestly desired to have an intelligent discussion of this disease and to consider some effective means to check its spread. This consultation was of singular importance, for it was this group of physicians, called together to protect the public from the ravages of the "throat distemper," who organized the first medical society in America. To the joint meeting in the Council Chamber they invited Dr. Simon Tufts, a leading physician of Medford and the surrounding country and whose practice extended as far as Haverhill and Newbury. Since the epidemic had already reached Newbury, Tufts could relate his own experiences and the information that he had received from the physicians who practised there. His Boston audience was undoubtedly amazed by the many astounding facts that he could tell about this new disease. There was that mysterious appearance in Kingston in homes four miles apart; there were other outbreaks in various places when there were no apparent contacts; the uncontrolled progress, the violent symptoms, and the unusually high mortality surely must have made his story all the more impressive. It was a time for very serious thought, because a dangerous enemy was about to attack the metropolis of New England. Perhaps this impending danger may have caused some uneasiness, but it did not cause despair for the Boston people had great confidence in their own physicians, and, as it later became quite evident, the physicians had no mean opinion of themselves. For some time they had secretly suspected that the "Eastern Distemper" had been so deadly only because the small town physicians, with limited training and experience, had neither recognized the disease nor prescribed the proper treatment. Thus they welcomed this opportunity to try the correct procedures, but after prolonged and thoughtful consideration of all the evidence and various defensive plans they were able to agree upon only one important point:— "That the said Distemper was communicated by means of a bad Air and not by Contagion." Of this, they were absolutely certain. There was hardly time to inform the people of this significant fact when great excitement prevailed among the physicians and fathers of the town. Within a week a serious situation had developed.

While the meeting was in progress, indeed, at the very moment when the "bad Air" theory was announced, a young man named How was on his way from Exeter to Boston. He was returning home to tell his widowed mother that during the recent Exeter epidemic a brother had been fatally stricken with a "Distemper in the Throat." A few days after he arrived at his home on Orange Street in the south end of the town he, too, complained of a sore throat and the famous Dr. Zabdiel Boylston was immediately consulted. Boylston recognized the dread disease at once, prescribed the customary pukes and purges, and proceeded to let some blood, but it appears from the records that for some unknown reason he failed to report the case. Some years before this, Boylston had been engaged in a heated controversy with most of his professional brethren and perhaps at this time he had no desire to cooperate in their plans or perhaps he thought that if the disease was not contagious then it was of no concern to others. Now, it was customary at that time "to watch o'er ourselves and one another," and somehow the Rev. Dr. Nathaniel Williams heard the news and immediately informed the selectmen of what was going on. Boylston was requested to appear at the Council Chamber and he then agreed that his patient had the same horrible disease that had been causing so much trouble in New Hampshire. That was all the selectmen wished to know and with that information they hastened to Justices Anthony Stoddard and Samuel Sewall and asked for a warrant to remove this patient to a pest-house on Spectacle Island.

It is not quite clear why they wanted to isolate the patient if the disease was not contagious, unless there were some doubts about the "bad Air" theory and an island seemed the safest place to test it out, but nevertheless they wanted him moved, and they wanted him moved quickly. The slightly bewildered justices, not appreciating the need for haste, advised the selectmen first to renovate the hospital and make it more comfortable for the reception of the sick. Obviously irritated by this delay, the selectmen went on with their plans with the utmost possible speed and dispatched "A Carpenter, a glazier and other hands" down to the island to complete the reconstruction. Meanwhile, arrangements were made with Dr. Hugh Kennedy to be resident physician and to care for all the patients who were expected to be quarantined. Within twenty-four hours from the time that Boylston's case was first reported, detailed preparations had been made for a serious and extensive epidemic. But in the best laid plans of the selectmen one very important item had been overlooked, for it seems that the request for a warrant was based upon a law that concerned only contagious cases and the physicians had already definitely stated that the distemper was not that kind of a disease. Dr. Boylston readily admitted that it was a serious disease, but at the same time insisted that his patient was not dangerous to others and apparently was not anxious to have him go. The worried selectmen, not yet convinced, decided to try other schemes and that same day they sent a committee consisting of John Jeffries Esq., Capt. Jonathan Armitage, and Capt. Forsyth to call on the widow How. They discussed the advantages of the hospital, stressed the dangers of an epidemic, and urged the widow to consider the other people in the town. These arguments proved ineffective, for the mother's love for her son was greater than her interest in the public health. She very decidedly refused, indeed, she defiantly told them that they could go and "Rase the Foundations of her House, before She would Suffer it." The selectmen, not anticipating all these obstacles to their plans, became more and more provoked and asked for a second warrant to break down the doors and forcibly remove the patient. The justices refused. The affair was brought to the attention of the Governor and Council who were unwilling to interfere and prudently referred the selectmen back to the justices of the peace. For the third and last time a warrant was requested. This time it would be granted, provided the physicians would only admit that the disease was spread by contact, but the physicians, of course, would agree to no such thing. So the selectmen, deciding upon a plan that did not require a warrant, "Ordered proper Persons to keep a Strict Watch at the said House, until further Order, to prevent any Communication with the same." Just as the controversy was concluded to the satisfaction of the contending parties, the patient died.[40]

It may have been the "watch" or an insufficient amount of "bad Air" or the state of grace in Boston or just pure good luck, but at any rate "No infection was observed to spread or catch in that Quarter of the Town." Meanwhile, during all the excitement about the warrants, some alarming rumors had reached the country towns that "Several Families" in Boston were suffering from the distemper, and the selectmen had then to worry about the effect upon the country trade. So they advertised in the newspapers[41] on October 23, that such reports were exaggerated and groundless "And That it is, thro' the Goodness of God, as healthy a Time as has been known for many years past."[40] This reassuring statement, however, no sooner appeared in print than an epidemic was discovered in many sections of the town. It had quietly begun the previous August, away up in the north end, and had made slow but steady progress during the succeeding months. The first cases had:

> ... *white specks in the Throat,* and a *cutaneous efflorescence*: A few more in the same Neighbourhood were seized in like manner, about the same time. Towards the end of *September* it appeared in several parts of the Town, with a complaint of *soreness in the Throat, Tonsils swelled and speckt, Uvula relaxed, slight Fever, flush in the Face,* and an *Erysipelas like efflorescence on the neck, chest and extremities*; but being of no fatal or bad consequence, nothing more than a common cold was suspected.[42]

[40] *Report of the Record Commissioners of the City of Boston containing the Records of the Boston Selectmen, 1716-1736.* Boston, 1885, 279 et seq. The patient was probably Israel Howe (Israel[3], Israel[2], Abraham[1]) b. Feb. 17, 1719; d. Oct. 10, 1735. (Howe Genealogies.)
[41] *Boston News-Letter,* Oct. 16-23, 1735.
[42] William Douglass: *Practical History* ... etc. Boston, 1736, 2.

At first the disease attracted very little attention, but by November it had become more prevalent and some of the patients died, with signs and symptoms that were somewhat similar to those observed in the How case. It then dawned upon the physicians that the dreadful "throat distemper" had actually invaded the town. Meanwhile, no new cases were seen in the vicinity of Orange Street, so the watch system of isolation was abandoned and other events seemed to confirm the previous opinion that the disease was caused by "some occult Quality in the Air." As winter approached it became readily apparent that a sizable epidemic was at hand and nothing could have helped more to spread the alarm than a doleful broadside which appeared about this time:[43]

A Lamentation

On the prevailing Sickness, in many Towsn in *New-England*, with an earnest Call to Young and Old, to turn from Sin, and to seek GOD's Face and Favour.

> Both Young and Old, come mourn with me,
>   with bitter Lamentation,
> Here is a Call from CHRIST above,
>   to th' rising Generation.

    *   *   *

> For GOD above, in Righteousness,
>   an Angel sent with Power,
> Who with a Sword already drawn
>   our Children to devour.

    *   *   *

> GOD smitten hath with sore Plagues,
>   our Children young and small,
> Which makes me weep exceedingly,
>   and on CHRIST's Name to call.

    *   *   *

> This mortal Plague doth much enrage,
>   among our little Bands,
> And sudden Death doth stop the Breath
>   of these our little Lambs.

---

[43] Broadside in the Mass. Hist. Soc. Although undated, the internal evidence places it about 1735-6.

A Lamentation

On the prevailing Sickness, in many Towns in *New-England*, with an earnest Call to Young and Old, to turn from Sin, and to seek GOD's Face and Favour.

BOTH Young and Old, come mourn with me,
 with bitter Lamentation,
Here is a Call from CHRIST above,
 to th' rising Generation.

For GOD above, in Righteousness,
 an Angel sent with Power,
Who with a Sword already drawn
 our Children to devour.

It makes my very Heart to bleed,
 and lye upon the Ground,
When I do hear our Children dear
 by sudden Death's abound.

GOD smitten hath with sore Plagues,
 our Children young and small,
Which makes we weep exceedingly,
 and on CHRIST's Name to call.

It makes me weep in sorrows deep,
 to hear the dying moan,
Which Death has made, in these our Days,
 among our little Ones.

This mortal Plague doth much corage,
 among our little Bands,
And sudden Death doth stop the Breath
 of these our little Lambs.

What mourning Sighs, and loud Out cries,
 comes from the Eastern Towns
Of Children crying, and others dying,
 which makes a doleful Sound.

What Tears apace, run from our Face,
 to hear our Children crying
For help from pain, but all in vain,
 we cannot help their dying.

My Pen and Heart I will impart
 to make this Declaration,
Of Children dying, and others crying,
 a sad and strange Relation.

They cry with pain, but all in vain,
 no succour can they find,
From Father, Mother, nor no other,
 for Death has them assign'd ——

This strange Disease doth mostly seize
 those that are young and tender,
And 'tis so smart, it strikes the Heart,
 and makes 'em to surrender.

O sad estate, and desperate,
 of these our little ones,
Who lye in pain, and so remain,
 they help can find from none.

The Doctor's Art, can find no part,
 nor Cure for this Distemper;
By Physick long, nor Cordials strong,
 they cannot find the Center.

It is unknown to any one
 and all the Doctors skill,
To cure this Plague, or to engage
 to cure it at their will.

They're in the dark, in every part,
 and cannot find it out,
From whence it strikes, and where it lights
 they cannot point it out.

If we should call the Doctors all
 and let them all engage,
We cannot find in any kind
 that they can cure this Plague.

If Doctors joyn, and do combine,
 to find out this Distemper,
They're in the dark in every part,
 and cannot find the Center.

We can't conceive, or do believe,
 that they were Sinners more
Then we have been, and lived in,
 O let us sin no more.

Let's search the Cause, 'tis breach of Laws,
 that punishes for Sin,
That brings down Plagues in every Age,
 as it has ever been.

Such Punishment is often sent,
 on Gospel-Light Offenders,
For GOD is just, and has profess'd,
 to punish such Transgressors.

GOD's holy Days, in many ways,
 we have not kept aright,
But have been slack, and turned back,
 against the Gospel Light.

Ungrateful Sins have ever been
 most odious in GOD's sight,
Then let's repent with one consent,
 and pray both Day and Night.

By sore Droughts and Pestilence
 we've had most awful Calls,
And likewise by most dreadful Wars,
 we've had great Warnings all.

The loudest Call we had of all,
 was by an Earthquake strong,
Which did us shake, and make us quake,
 and from our Sins refrain.

New-England's Sins have greater been
 than Sins of Heathen round,
Such breach of Laws, is the grand Cause,
 GOD's Judgments do abound.

Let's go alone, and pray each one,
 and turn from all Transgression,
With holy love to GOD above,
 and turn from all Oppression.

Young Men and Maids, let me perswade
 you to a Reformation,
For this loud Call is to you all,
 of rising Generation.

Let Holiness your Souls possess,
 serve GOD while you are young,
In early Days, live to GOD's Praise
 and CHRIST will be your own.

In youthful Days, live to GOD's Praise
 whilst you are young and tender,
And CHRIST will own, and GOD alone,
 will of your Lives be tender.

Come let us all, both great and small,
 both Young and Old together,
Turn to the LORD with one accord,
 and mourn for Sin for ever.

(Courtesy of the Massachusetts Historical Society.)

> What tears apace, run from our Face,
>   to hear our Children crying
> For help from pain, but all in vain,
>   we cannot help their dying.
>
> *   *   *
>
> *New England's* Sins have greater been
>   than Sins of Heathen round,
> Such breach of Laws, is the grand Cause,
>   GOD's Judgments do abound.
>
> *   *   *
>
> Come let us all, both great and small,
>   both Young and Old together,
> Turn to the Lord with one accord,
>   and mourn for Sin for ever.

The weather was not as cold as usual, but a constant disagreeable chill in the air added to the discomfort. The severity of the disease also seemed to increase and the weekly Journal of Burials disclosed more and more deaths. Near the end of December the Governor proclaimed that Thursday the eighth of January was to be:

> ... A Day of solemn Prayer and Humiliation with Fasting, thro'out this Province on account of the unusual, malignant and mortal Distemper, wherewith several Towns within this Province are visited, and by which great Numbers, especially of the younger People, have been removed by Death; there being great Danger that the said Sickness will become more epidemical.[44]

This proclamation was read in many churches throughout the province.[45] In February there was another proclamation:

> Upon consideration of the holy Anger of Almighty God evidently manifested in the various Judgments inflicted on us (more especially in sending us a mortal Sickness, which has already greatly wasted our numbers, and threatens yet more terrible Effects, unless prevented by the merciful Interposition of Providence;) ...

---

[44] *Boston News-Letter*, Dec. 18-25, 1735.

[45] "On Dec. 28, 1735, Mr. Dunbar read a proclamation on the matter of an unusual and malignant distemper in many towns of the province, which was likely to spread through the land."—D. T. V. Huntoon: *Hist. of Canton*, p. 180; also Timothy Orne of Salem entered in his diary: "Generall Fast for the Distemper @ the Eastward." Ms. in Essex Institute.

By His EXCELLENCY
JONATHAN BELCHER, Esq;
Captain General and Governour in Chief in and over His Majesty's Province of the *Massachusetts-Bay* in *New-England*.

A Proclamation for a general FAST.

UPON Consideration of the holy Anger of Almighty GOD evidently manifested in the various Judgments inflicted on us (more especially in sending among us a *mortal Sickness*, which has already greatly wasted our Numbers, and threatens yet more terrible Effects, unless prevented by the merciful Interposition of Providence;) upon Consideration likewise of our absolute Dependence on the Blessing of GOD for Success in the Interests and Affairs of the Spring and Summer ensuing;

I have thought fit, with the Advice of His Majesty's Council, to order and appoint Thursday the First Day of *April* next to be observed as a Day of solemn *Fasting* and *Prayer* throughout this Province, hereby exhorting both Ministers and People religiously to attend the Duties of the said Day, by sincere and penitent Confession of their manifold Sins, whereby GOD hath been provoked to visit this People with sore and grievous Calamities; and by humble and earnest Supplications to the GOD of all Grace for averting the Tokens of his righteous Displeasure and conferring on us all needful Favours: In particular, That he would long preserve the Life of our Sovereign Lord the KING and our most gracious QUEEN, together with his Royal highness the Prince of Wales, the Duke, and the other Branches of the Royal Family; That he would grant his merciful Influence & Conduct to his Majesty's Councils for the Continuance of the Peace of his Kingdoms and Dominions, and for the restoring of Peace to *Europe*, under his Majesty's wise Mediation; That he would please to direct and bless the Administration of the Government of this Province; That he would give us a favourable Seeds-Time, and in due Season a plentiful Harvest; That he would prosper our Trade and Navigation, and maintain the Peace of our Sea-Coasts and Inland-Borders; and that he would compassionate our great Distress under the wasting and mortal Sickness, by sanctifying this awful Visitation and restoring to us the Voice of Health; And above all, That he would grant unto us the plentiful Effusions of the *HOLY SPIRIT*, that the Sense of his righteous Displeasure against us may effect a general Repentance and Reformation throughout the Whole Land, and that the Kingdom of our Lord and Saviour JESUS CHRIST may come, and the whole Earth be filled with his Glory: And all servile Labour and Recreations are hereby forbidden on said Day.

Given at the Council Chamber in *Boston*, the Twenty-fifth Day of *February*, 1736, in the Ninth Year of the Reign of Our Sovereign Lord GEORGE the Second, by the Grace of GOD, of *Great-Britain, France* and *Ireland*, KING, Defender of the Faith, &c.

By His Excellency's Command,
with the Advice of the Council,
J. Willard, Secr.

J. BELCHER.

GOD save the KING.

BOSTON: Printed by J. Draper, Printer to His Excellency the GOVERNOUR and COUNCIL.

(Courtesy of the American Antiquarian Society.)

Meanwhile, the Medical Society attacked their problem in true scientific fashion and made every effort to control this apparently new disease which was rapidly spreading throughout the town. They sent letters to some of the better known country doctors and requested specific answers to many questions. More information was wanted about the nature of this terrible disease, its various appearances, its usual course, and its most common complications. And a little while later they inserted the same questions in the newspapers[46] requesting replies from any or all physicians who desired "to furnish their Mite, for the Good of the Publick . . . towards the History and Cure of the Epidemical Sore Throats, which at present prevail in New-England."

Either from the answers that were received or from the newspaper accounts it was learned that as yet no effectual remedy had been found and that the epidemic was still raging in the "Eastward" towns. From Hampton Falls, Dover, Portsmouth, and Newbury, the reports were all the same—many families losing all their children—and it was feared that similar catastrophes would soon occur in Boston. But in spite of the rapid spread of the disease some favorable and unexpected turn took place, and most of the Boston children quickly recovered from their illnesses. The mortality was not nearly so great as had been anticipated and recoveries occurred as quickly as anyone had even dared to wish. Now, why a disease that had been so frightful in New Hampshire should be so surprisingly mild in Boston was not difficult for the Boston doctors to explain. After all, it was perfectly obvious to anyone that superior medical ability had finally solved the problem and brought forth an effectual treatment. One kind soul, who "out of pity to his fellow Creatures, was willing to communicate his Judgment and Experience," and who was also very clever with a lancet, intimated that the country doctors had not opened the proper veins, so he wrote to the *Boston Gazette*:

Method of Cure of Throat Distemper . . . First be sure than a vein be opened under the tongue, and if that can't be done, open a vein in the arm, which must be first done, or all other means will be ineffectual. Then take borax or honey to bathe or anoint the mouth and throat, and lay on the Throat a plaister Unguintum Dialthae. . . . I have known many other things used, especially a root called Physick Root, filarie, or five-leaved

---

[46] *Boston News-Letter*, Feb. 12-19, 1736; *Boston Weekly Post-Boy*, Feb. 16, 1735/6.

physick; also a root that I know no name for, only Canker Root. But be sure and let blood, and that under the tongue. . . .[47]

There were other Boston doctors, however, who held slightly different opinions because they had seen many patients recover without recourse to bleeding, so they concluded that the country doctors had probably bled their patients to death. Some explanation was indeed necessary for the higher mortality in the "Eastward" towns; obviously there must have been some fault in the treatment used by the country doctors. The Boston public were told on the front pages of their newspapers that these small-town physicians "altho' their bad Success evidently shews that they have no manner of Notion of the Nature of the Disease or Method of Cure yet persist in one invariable Method to kill very successfully, *secundum Artem*." Regardless of the various explanations, the fact remained that the "throat distemper" as it appeared in Boston was much more easily cured.

Although the frightening suspense was greatly relieved, the epidemic continued to spread and reached a peak in March, when during the second week there were twenty-four burials. A month later neighboring governments were still apprehensive that the distemper was carried by goods, and they had so restricted their Boston trade that the selectmen again summoned the physicians and requested their written opinion about the spread of the disease. It was voted to publish the comforting news:[48]

Boston 24 April 1736

The *Select-men of the Town of Boston*, in order to inform the Trading Part of our neighbouring *Colonies*, concerning the state of the present *prevailing Distemper* in this Place, did desire a Meeting of as many *Practitioners in Physick* as could then be conveniently obtained. The *Practitioners* being accordingly met, did unanimously agree to the following Articles:

1. That upon the first appearance of this *Illness* in *Boston* the *Select-men* did advise with the Practitioners; but they at that time having not had opportunities of observing the Progress of the *Distemper*, it was thought

---

[47] *Boston Gazette*—copy in *New York Weekly Journal*, March 8, 1735/6. Signed by N. H.

[48] *Boston Weekly News-Letter*, April 22-29, 1736. *Report of the Record Commissioners of the City of Boston, containing the Records of the Boston Selectmen*, 1716-1736. Boston, 1885, 294.

advisable (until further experience) to shut up that *Person* who was supposed to have received it in *Exeter* to the Eastward, upon his death the Watch was soon removed, but no infection was observed to spread in that quarter of the Town; therefore, no watches were appointed in the other Parts of the Town where it afterwards appeared, the Practitioners judging it to proceed from some occult *Quality in the Air*, and not from any observable *Infection* communicated *by Persons or Goods*.

2. *The Practitioners* and their Families have not been seized with this Distemper in a more *remarkable* manner (and as it happened not so much) than other Families in Town, even than those Families who live in solitary Parts thereof.

3. As to the Mortality or Malignity of this Distemper, all whom it may concern are referred to the Boston Weekly Journal of Burials; by the *Burials* it is notorious, that scarce any Distemper, even the most favourable which has at any Time prevailed so generally, has produced fewer deaths.

4. As formerly, so now again after many Months Observations, we conclude, That the present prevailing Distemper appears to us to *proceed from some Affection of the Air, and not from any personal Infection received from the sick, or Goods in their neighbourhood.*

Nathaniel Williams
William Douglass
John Cutler
Hugh Kennedy
William Davis
Thomas Bulfinch.

Although the number of deaths continued to decrease, some excitement still prevailed, and on May 11, 1736, another fast was held at the Old North Church "for the benefit of the rising generation."[49] When the epidemic was over it was supposed that about one-fourth of all the people in Boston had contracted the disease, and that out of the four thousand cases one hundred and fourteen had died.

V

THE DIAGNOSIS

> If Doctors joyn, and do combine,
> to find out this Distemper,
> They're in the dark in every part,
> and cannot find the Center.
> —A Lamentation.

---

[49] A. E. Bates: Almanac Notes, in *Old Northwest Quarterly*, Oct., 1907, 348.

In July, 1736, when the epidemic was "almost over," William Douglass (1691-1752) published *The Practical HISTORY of A New Epidemical Eruptive Miliary Fever, with an Angina Ulcusculosa which Prevailed in Boston New-England in the Years 1735 and 1736.*

William Douglass was born in Scotland, received a good medical education abroad, came to Boston about 1716, acquired a very successful practice, and for a long time was the only physician in Boston with a medical degree. If some of his biographers are correct, however, he was an irresponsible person never to be trusted. This suggests that his character be considered in somewhat more detail, because the exact diagnosis of the "throat distemper" depends in some measure upon his works. Early in his career, when the controversy about inoculation was at its height, Douglass had quarrelled with Cotton Mather and the clergy, for whom he had no respect. He was probably a little jealous when he doubted that the clergy were qualified to discuss purely medical subjects; nevertheless, he very rightly maintained that inoculation was a dangerous procedure, especially when haphazardly performed. He had an unfortunate way of expressing his opinions and long after the quarrel was over made enemies of those religiously inclined, and it was chiefly because of this disrespect for personalities and conventions that most of his biographers have had little respect for him. One said that he was "a scamp, perhaps, certainly a liar," and even a modern student of eighteenth century religious thought describes him as "a deist with a bitter contempt for revivalism—on all subjects a most partial and inaccurate writer."

Douglass also wrote a *Summary, Historical and Political of . . . the British Settlements in North America*, and after a study based chiefly upon this work, another biographer wrote:

He was a man of large but heterogeneous knowledge, and blessed with a sovereign confidence in himself and his own opinions; and being also dogmatic, intolerant, of quick temper and boundless energy, fiery as a friend, still more fiery as an enemy, fond of strife, glib in speech, with a passion for rushing into print, his life was one prolonged and blissful warfare with all persons whom he could pick a quarrel with,—chiefly, his own professional brethren, likewise the clergy, the magistrates, and the successive governors of the colony.[50]

---

[50] Moses C. Tyler: *Hist. of Amer. Literature*, 1879, ii, 151.

With this information about the man, one hesitates to trust his descriptions of the disease, but fortunately Dr. G. H. Weaver, another biographer, has considered Douglass' many contributions to medicine and science and presented him in an entirely different light.[51] Douglass was intensely interested in botany, earthquakes, the weather, maps, and public school education. His criticisms of contemporary physicians, especially the quacks, were written in an effort to place the practice of medicine upon a higher plane. His studies on inflated currency make interesting reading at the present time. Weaver further describes him:

> ... he was the first really remarkable medical man in this country. He was a widely educated and skillful physician and his writings were a real addition to the literature of the world ... Aside from his medical interests we must recognize in William Douglass a man of encyclopedic knowledge, of prodigious energy and perseverance, interested in all lines of scientific and human activity, a fearless public-spirited citizen, and an economist of high grade. It is time that we should recognize him as a man for any time and place, and should honor him for achievements accomplished under most adverse surroundings.

To any fair-minded reader the disease descriptions in the *Practical History* are ample proof that with all his faults William Douglass was capable of keen clinical observation. He describes in minute detail a typical case with onset, course, and treatment, and also some unusual varieties of the disease. One can almost make a diagnosis from the complications which he mentions. Those who are familiar with eighteenth century medical publications readily recognize this work as one of unusual merit and it deserves to be known as an American medical classic. Dr. Weaver, an authority on the disease, says that "it was the first adequate clinical description of scarlet fever in English ... It seems impossible that any doubt could arise regarding the identity in the minds of any one who has read Douglass' description and is familiar with the disease." So we need not look beyond Douglass' *Practical History* for a diagnosis. There was an epidemic of scarlet fever in Boston during 1735-36.

But was it scarlet fever that was raging in New Hampshire? Douglass said:—"There is no Symptom, even the most malignant that has appeared in New Hampshire, but what the like has occurred

---

[51] George H. Weaver: *Life and Writings of William Douglass.* Bull. Soc. Med. Hist. of Chicago. April, 1921, xi, 229-59.

in Boston." He was certain that the two epidemics were caused by the same disease. This conclusion seemed warranted, for here in New England was an apparently new disease; here was an apparent contact (the How case) between Exeter and Boston; here was an epidemic that started in the country and spread swiftly from town to town and reached Boston about the time it was expected; and in both New Hampshire and Boston children were the victims and sore throat was the chief complaint. Medical historians agree that it was an epidemic of a single disease, but they differ in opinions of the diagnosis. Creighton,[52] Weaver,[53] and others have considered this to be the first great epidemic of scarlet fever in this country, but on the other hand, Jacobi,[54]

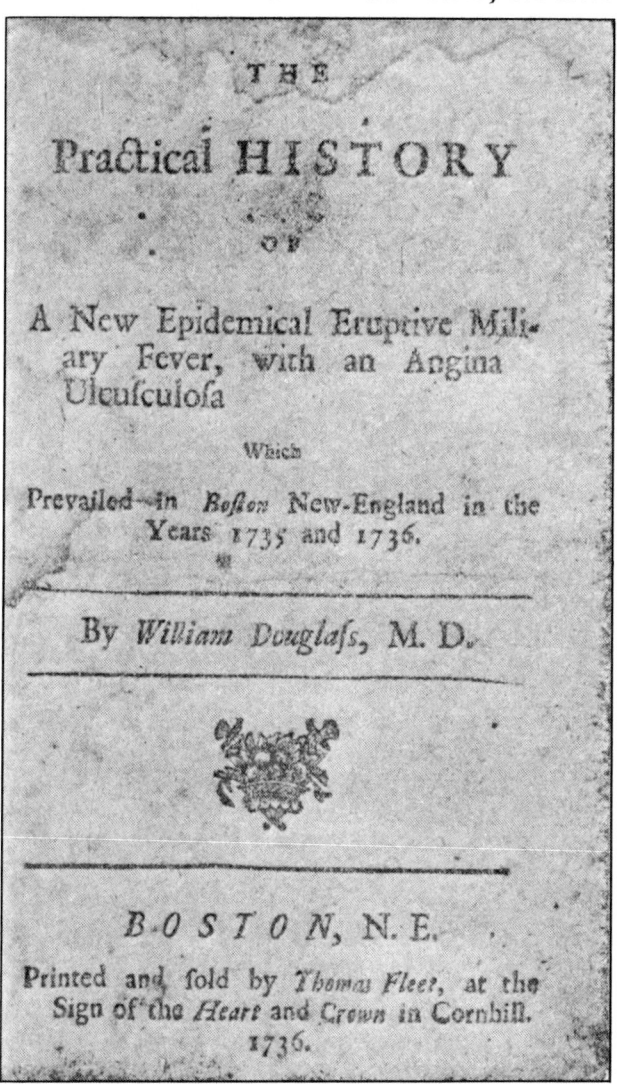

(Courtesy of the Massachusetts Historical Society.)

---
[52] Charles Creighton: *Hist. of Epidemics in Britain.* 1894, ii, 685.
[53] G. H. Weaver: Scarlet Fever, *Abt's Pediatrics.* 1925, vi, 298.
[54] Abraham Jacobi: *A Treatise on Diphtheria.* 1880, 4.

Packard,[55] and others have considered it to be diphtheria. Samuel A. Green wrote:[56] "It has been considered also to be scarlatina; but the description leaves little doubt in my mind that the diagnosis at the present time would be diphtheria." My own opinion is that neither scarlet fever nor diphtheria adequately explains the epidemic as a whole and that, heretofore, the diagnosis has rested upon incomplete evidence. It seems that the scarlet fever advocates have put too much emphasis on Douglass and that the diphtheria advocates have not given him sufficient consideration. I hope to prove that at the time of the Boston scarlet fever epidemic, diphtheria was raging in New Hampshire.

If this conception of the epidemic is correct, it may seem strange that Douglass should have given an accurate, detailed, clinical account and yet have drawn a false conclusion. The explanation is found in his own words. His account of scarlet fever is valuable because it was founded upon personal observation:

> This is a Real History of the distemper as it appeared in Boston New England, taken clinically from life and not copied. There is no stroak or clause, but what I can vouch by real not imaginary cases. It is founded only upon observation or phenomina, that is upon the Symptoms that appeared in the course of this Epidemical disease; it must therefore be of permanent truth.

So far, so good; there was no chance for error so long as he described exactly what he saw. But he admits, and this is the point that has been overlooked, that his information about the New Hampshire epidemic was obtained from others—or to quote him—"as we were informed." It is probable that he received most of his information from the answers to his newspaper questionnaire[57] or from Dr. Tufts at that first meeting of the Boston physicians on October 1, 1735.

Douglass travelled about New England to obtain material for his maps and botanical studies, but there is no evidence that he went to New Hampshire during the epidemic. There is good reason to believe that he did not go; he was a very busy practitioner and had more than he could do in Boston. Though it is begging the question somewhat, I firmly believe that Douglass, with his keen clinical sense, would have readily seen the difference in the diseases had he

---

[55] Packard: *Hist. of Med. in United States.* 1931, vol. i.

[56] Green: *History of Medicine in Massachusetts.* 1881, 69.

[57] *Boston Weekly News-Letter*, Feb. 12-19, 1736. On account of the similarity of many expressions in this questionnaire, and in the *Practical History* I believe that Douglass very probably composed most of it.

actually gone to New Hampshire. As a matter of fact, he did go to some of the neighboring towns at a later time and it is significant that following these personal observations, he wrote another somewhat different clinical account. The error does not make the *Practical History* a less creditable performance, for original disease descriptions are of utmost importance in man's warfare against disease. Medicine will always be indebted to William Douglass,— he was a valuable spy who went into the enemy's camp and returned with a description of his position and his numbers. Nevertheless, it is important to realize that the two diseases were confused, since it partly explains why scarlet fever and diphtheria were considered the same disease for many years.

The diagnosis of the New Hampshire epidemic has been surmised by many historians, but very few have offered supporting facts or reasons. The histories of the separate towns seldom yield enough information to make an exact diagnosis, but sufficient material concerning the whole epidemic is now available to support a diagnosis that leaves little room for doubt. The New Hampshire disease had four primary characteristics. It was a very fatal, childhood, epidemic disease that chiefly affected the throat, and therefore could not have been measles, influenza, smallpox, dysentery, or any other disease that does not satisfy the definition. Diphtheria, scarlet fever, and septic (or streptococcic) sore throat are the only diseases that need to be seriously considered. The last is regarded by some clinicians as fundamentally the same as scarlet fever but without a rash. It attacks adults as well as children and in epidemic form is generally caused by a contaminated milk supply. Now, in Boston and the larger towns many families may have received their milk from one supply, but in the smaller country towns almost every family had its own supply. For these reasons the diagnosis of streptococcic sore throat seems to be improbable, and for practical purposes only the first two diseases need be considered.

For the benefit of the non-medical reader, it may be said that on paper, at least, scarlet fever and diphtheria are similar diseases. They frequently occur in epidemic form, have a tendency to attack the same age group—children under twenty years—and are characterized by sore throat and fever. Swallowing and breathing may be difficult in both diseases. Indeed, it is sometimes difficult to distinguish the two diseases by the appearance of the throat alone. In the great majority of cases, however, diphtheria begins insidiously, has no rash, and is accompanied, if untreated, by a very high mortality; scarlet fever begins suddenly, generally with vomiting, has a very distinct rash over most of the body, and, although it may be a very malignant disease in some epidemics, is usually less fatal than is diphtheria. It has already been stated that the disease in Boston was scarlet fever and now an attempt will be made to prove that the New Hampshire disease could not have been the same.

The fatality rate of a disease, or the number of deaths that occur in each one hundred cases, is frequently used, especially during epidemics, to compare different diseases or the same disease under different circumstances. Although it is seldom used for diagnostic purposes because of possible variations in the rate depending upon many complicating factors, it is of considerable value when applied to different phases of the "throat distemper" epidemic. Only a crude estimate can be made of the fatality rate of the New Hampshire and "Eastward" cases, as there are no available statistics of the number who recovered. Many were "brought down to the Brink of the Grave"; many had the disease "in a moderate Degree";[58] undoubtedly many were unaware of their infection. It was said that in some of the New Hampshire towns the fatality rate was "1 in 3 of the sick, in others 1 in 4, in scarce any fewer than 1 in 6."[59] At Kingston,[60] Scarborough,[61] and Presumscot Falls[62] there were short periods when the fatality approached one hundred per cent. A closer estimate can be made from a tabulation of the Hampton Falls records:

Ages	% of population	Population	Deaths	Fatality minimum
Under 10	32.1	404	160	39.6
10-20	24.6	310	40	12.9
Under 20	56.7	714	200	28.0
Over 20	43.3	546	10	1.8
Total	100.0	1260	210	15.2

Fitch counted 210 deaths, which he said was about one-sixth of the total population. With the aid of some New England eighteenth century census figures[63] we may suppose that there were

---
[58] Jabez Fitch: *An Account of the Numbers* . . . p. 11.
[59] William Douglass: *A Practical History* . . . p. 3.
[60] Ibid, 1.
[61] *Journal of the Rev. Thomas Smith.* Oct. 13, 1737.
[62] Ibid. Aug. 16, 1738.
[63] *Account of the Number of Inhabitants in the Colony of Connecticut, Jan. 1st, 1774.* Hartford, 1774.

about 714 children under 20 years of age, and if we further suppose that *every one* of them contracted the disease, then the *minimum* fatality rate was 28 per cent for this age group. In the group under 10 years of age there were about 404 children with a *minimum* fatality rate of 39.6 per cent. Let us suppose that only one-fourth of all the children under ten escaped the disease, either because they were immune or not exposed during the first year of the epidemic, then, of the remaining 303 children, 160 died which would give a fatality rate of 53 per cent. Although this is a crude method upon which to base conclusions, I believe that it does show that the *actual* fatality rate in Hampton Falls was very high, and probably near 60 per cent. Taking all available sources into consideration, the fatality rate of the "Eastward" cases can be roughly estimated at between 16^{64} and 60 per cent.

In comparison, the Boston epidemic was very mild indeed. Douglass said: "It is generally in so considerable a degree more favourable in Boston, than in the Townships where it first prevailed; that many can scarce be persuaded of its being the same Distemper." He compared the number of deaths during certain months of the winter and spring of 1735-36 with the number of deaths during the same months of previous healthy years, and computed that the epidemic was responsible for one hundred and fourteen deaths. He estimated that there were about four thousand cases of sickness, which would place the fatality rate at 2.8 per cent. Another observer[65] of the Boston epidemic said: ". . . I believe that not one to sixty Dies thereof . . ." This would give a fatality rate of 1.7 per cent. Although these also are crude estimates, they disclose beyond doubt that the Boston epidemic was very mild compared with the one in New Hampshire.

It is interesting to compare these figures with more recent ones. For diphtheria statistics one must go back to pre-antitoxin days, and as that was the time when the diagnosis rested upon clinical evidence alone, the figures are not strictly accurate and therefore the comparison is questionable. Nevertheless, of forty thousand cases of diphtheria in New York and Boston during the years 1880 to 1887,

---

[64] This is the lowest contemporary estimate of the "Eastward" fatality rate that I can find. It is taken from the works of William Douglass, who, I believe, confused the two diseases and therefore it may be the figure for some Massachusetts town where there were epidemics of both diseases. Nevertheless, I have included it in the New Hampshire figures.

[65] Signed "N. H." in *New York Weekly Journal*, March 8, 1735/6.

the fatality rate varied from 26 to 49 per cent.[66] For a number of years the scarlet fever fatality rate has steadily decreased. Seldom has it been over 30 per cent; the rate in eight American cities with over 500,000 cases from 1873 to 1913 was about 10 per cent;[67] the Connecticut rate from 1895 to 1929 varied from 6.6 per cent to 0.6 per cent, with an average five-year-period rate of 3.2 per cent.[68] To summarize these figures on fatality rates:

	Scarlet Fever	Diphtheria
Boston 1735-1736	1.7–2.8	
Connecticut 1895-1929	3.2	
Boston & New York 1880-1887		26–49
New Hampshire[69] 1735-1738		16–60

These figures indicate that diphtheria was the probable cause of the New Hampshire epidemic. Indeed, the fatality rate of untreated diphtheria could not possibly be under three per cent and the fatality rate of scarlet fever has never approached sixty per cent. If the fatality rates of the "throat distemper" are at all accurate, it is certain that two different diseases were present.

The death-rate, or the number of deaths in proportion to the population, is also used to compare diseases, especially during epidemics. Fitch estimated that in Hampton Falls one-sixth of the population died, which is at the rate of 166.6 for each one thousand people. In Byfield, Mass., one-seventh of the population died. The population of Kingston in 1735 was probably less than a thousand, and so the estimated death-rate is over 100. Apparently the rate was somewhat less in Portsmouth, Exeter, and other places, but slightly more in Haverhill. The total population of New Hampshire has been estimated at 20,000 and by actual count there were about 1000 fatal cases during the first year of the epidemic (July 1, 1735-July 1, 1736). This rate of 50 deaths for each one thousand people depends upon the accuracy of the population estimates and upon the accuracy of the diagnosis in Fitch's series, nevertheless it is in striking contrast to the estimated death-rate for Boston, where, during the same period, there were 114 deaths among 16,000 people, or a rate of 7.1 deaths for each one thousand people. Some objection may be raised to this comparison of death-

---

[66] Billington and O'Dwyer: *Diphtheria*. 1899, 139.
[67] Donnally: Quoted by Weaver in *Abt's Pediatrics*. Art: Scarlet Fever.
[68] *Conn. Health Bulletin.* 1932, xlvi, 214.
[69] Including other "Eastward" towns.

rates because it is thought that epidemic diseases behave differently in rural and urban populations, nevertheless the difference is too great to be overlooked and has additional importance when taken with the other facts.

Some students readily admit that the New Hampshire epidemic was more severe, but they still believe that it was the same disease and that it became milder as it invaded Boston. This conclusion is based on the theory that epidemics may be very severe at first and become milder as time goes on. This supposition does not explain other facts. The epidemic was severe in Haverhill at nearly the same time that it was mild in Boston; it was severe in Marblehead in 1737, which was after the Boston epidemic had quieted down. As will be shown later, some towns had two epidemics, one more serious than the other, and it is extremely difficult to explain such facts on the assumption that one disease could show such variations.

Although occasionally found in very old genealogical and church records, multiple deaths are more frequently found during and after 1735, and most of them can be attributed to the "throat distemper." The term "multiple deaths" is here used to mean the deaths of two or more children of the same family within approximately one month. I believe that they have considerable diagnostic significance in separating the two diseases comprising the epidemic, because such deaths are characteristic of the disease in New Hampshire and other "Eastward" towns. A few of the countless instances have already been given, but here the family record of John and Jemima Boynton of Newbury will serve as an extreme but not unique example:

Mary Boynton	died	"	December 20	1735
Sarah	"	"	December 20	1735
John	"	"	December 21	1735
William	"	"	December 21	1735
David	"	"	December 26	1735
Francis	"	"	December 26	1735
Samuel	"	"	January 4	1735/6
Jemima	"	"	February 11	1735/6

I do not believe that scarlet fever caused these deaths. At the present time, at least, that disease seldom causes two deaths in the same family. Even in the days when the scarlet fever fatality rate was said to be 20 to 30 per cent, it would seem improbable that in a family of eight or ten children all would get the disease, and, if they did, also improbable that more than two or three would die.

Moreover, scarlet fever deaths generally occur as a result of complications and the six to eight deaths in the same family would probably be spread over a longer period of time. It is said, however, that during some epidemics scarlet fever has been known to cause many deaths in many families. Osler mentions the deaths in rapid succession of four or five members of a family as an illustration of family susceptibility to the disease. The *Vital Records* of many Massachusetts towns show multiple deaths between 1839 and 1850, and the diagnosis is given as "scarlet fever." So, for the present, it is admitted that scarlet fever can be very severe in certain epidemics and that it has caused multiple deaths in the past, but all the available evidence indicates that scarlet fever during 1735-40 was not very much more serious than it is today and therefore was incapable of causing repeated multiple deaths. The figures given by two independent observers of the large Boston epidemic show conclusively that it was a comparatively mild disease and there is additional evidence that it was mild in other towns. Also, it must be evident that with only 114 deaths out of 4000 cases, there could not have been many instances of multiple deaths during the Boston epidemic. Douglass mentions that multiple deaths occurred in the "Eastward" towns, but neglects to say that they occurred in Boston. Therefore, during the time of the "throat distemper" epidemic (1735-40), if frequent and extreme examples of multiple deaths can be found, I believe that the diagnosis of diphtheria is justified. On the other hand, the occurrence of two, three, or four deaths in a *single* family has no significant diagnostic value.

In addition to the marked differences revealed by death-rates, fatality rates, and multiple deaths, there are differences in the clinical descriptions of the New Hampshire and Boston epidemics. One must be cautious in the selection of material. Most historians of the New Hampshire and Maine towns describe a disease that resembles scarlet fever, but the similarity in wording and phraseology show that these historians, almost without exception, have copied their material from a common source—Belknap's *History of New Hampshire*. Belknap, writing in 1791, obtained his information from William Douglass' *Practical History*, so the descriptions apply not to the New Hampshire epidemic at all but only to the Boston cases. Therefore, one cannot rely upon nineteenth century histories and must admit only contemporary evidence.

The most important and complete description of the "Eastward" cases appeared in the *Boston Gazette*. The particular issue does not seem to be extant, but the description was copied by the publisher of the *New York Gazette* (Feb. 17-24, 1735/6). Although originally published in Boston, the writer definitely says that his description applies to the New Hampshire epidemic:

No Disease has never raved in *New England* (except the Small-Pox) which has struck such an universal Terror into People, as that which has lately visited *Kingston, Exeter Hampton* and other Parts of the Province of *New-Hampshire,* and tho' something has been divers Times said of it in the publick News Papers, it yet wants a Name. It has been among young People and Children, pretty universal and very mortal; but what surprizes me most is, that the Physicians in those Parts (altho' their bad Success evidently shews that they have no manner of Notion of the Nature of the Disease or Method of Cure) yet persist in one invariable Method to kill very successfully, *secundum Artem*. This Disease invades generally such as are very young, but they feel at the first somewhat listless and heavy for a Day or two, and then begin to complain of a Soreness in the Throat, and if you look into the Motion you'l discover upon the Uvula and Parts adjacent the Cuticula raised in Spots of different Sizes, sometimes to a quarter of an Inch Diameter, and fill'd with a laudable coloured Pus. This is the pathognomonick Sign of the Disease. In a Day or two more, they have the same Cough as in the common humorous Quinzey; the next Day a Fever rises, and the Cough is often between whiles very loose; the Patient now begins to breath hard, and almost loses his Voice, being able only to whisper; and a Day more makes (with Coughing) only a whistling kind of Noise, and the next Day pays his Debt to Nature. These are the different Stages of the Disease, which, as the Disease is more or less fierce, are longer or shorter. . . .

This article, which appeared at very nearly the same time as Douglass' account of the Boston epidemic, not only establishes the diagnosis of the New Hampshire epidemic, but it is the first printed description of unquestionable diphtheria to appear in America. In it, as in other accounts of the "Eastward" cases, no mention is made of any rash, whereas in the Boston epidemic the rash was the most significant finding, as is shown by the title of Douglass' *Practical History*. Moreover, Douglass himself stated that in New Hampshire the eruption was "noticeable only in a few, and in these it was called a Scarlet Fever." This statement supports my thesis but, unfortunately, it is not a first-hand description, for, as I have said before, Douglass probably obtained his information about the New Hampshire cases from someone else.

The Kingston church records state that "This mortality was By

Numb. 538

THE
New-York Gazette

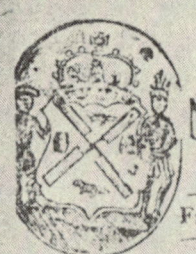 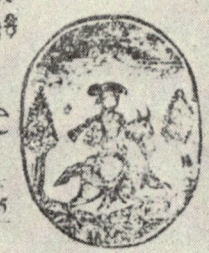

From Tuesday *February* 17. to *February* 24. 1735.

As several who have heard of the New-Distemper in the East Parts of New-England, are desirous to know something of the the Nature of it for their Satisfaction we publish the following Piece from the Boston Gazette.

NO Disease has never raved in *New-England* (except the Small-Pox) which has struck such an universal Terror into People, as that which has lately visited *Kingston, Exeter Hampton* and other Parts of the Province of *New-Hampshire*, and tho' something has been divers Times said of it in the publick News Papers, it yet wants a Name. It has been among young People and Children, pretty universal and very mortal; but what surprizes me most is, that the Physicians in those Parts (altho' their bad Success evidently shews that they have no manner of Notion of the Nature of the Disease or Method of Cure) yet persist in one invariable Method to kill very successfully, *secundum Artem.* This Disease invades generally such as are very young, but they feel at the first somewhat listless and heavy for a Day or two, and then begin to complain of a Soreness in the Throat, and if you then look into the Motion you'l discover upon the Uvula and Parts adjacent the Cuticula raised in Spots of different Sizes, sometimes to a quarter of an Inch Diameter, and fill'd with a Laudable coloured Pus. This is the pathognomonick Sign of the Disease. In a Day or two more, they have the same Cough as in the common humorous Quinzey; the next Day a Fever rises, and the Cough is often between whiles very loose; the Patient now begins to breath hard, and almost loses his Voice, being able only to whisper; and a Day more makes (with Coughing) only a whistling kind of Noise, and the next Day pays his Debt to Nature. These are the different Stages of the Disease, which, as the Disease is more or less fierce, are longer or shorter.

It sometimes begins with small Excoriations behind the Ears, which increase to a great Bigness (with swelling sometimes so large as to meet on the Forehead. In this Case the Patient is sometimes blind with it.

In others the parotid Glands are tumefied and exulcerate, so the Axillary, but the Inguinal rarely.

Oftentimes Tumours arise like a small Boil, break and spread to 5 or 6 Inches Diameter; these affect chiefly the hinder Part of the Head and Neck, between the Shoulders, the Back. &c.

When the Sores turn l ved or purple, Death is at hand. Many have the Tumour and sores who have no Sign of the Disease in the Throat, and vice versa.

Upon breathing a Vein (which by the bye in this Disease, is a pernicious Practice in general) the Texture of the Blood appears to be much broken.

A Fever arising is a good Symptom. A Strangury often arises from the Method of Cure, and which is pretty easily obviated.

Blisters to the Neck or Arms generally prove fatal, it being almost impossible to heal them; and no Wonder.

When they recover, they are a long time generally in getting well.

They very frequently die within 4 or 5 Days after the first Seizure, but rarely sooner, and sometimes after 15 Days.

The Indications to be satisfied in this Disease are many, and sometimes coincide.

I thought proper to give these few loose Hints of this Disease to the Publick, that they may have some true Information of it, and that the Physicians in the Country may have time to employ their Tho'ts upon it, not knowing but it may become so general, as sooner or later, to employ the most we have.

I am, SIR, Your humble Servant,
ÆSCULAPIUS.

An ODE for the 30th of January, w'ich should have been inserted before,

BLest Martyr, for whose Fate,
And our fore-Fathers Crimes we weep,
And still the sad Memorial keep,
From blest abodes cou'dst thou look down,
Thou wou'dst with pity own
Thy Britain's sufferings, as her guilt, are great
Twice eight hundred years before.
Like thee, by his Subjects try'd,
A Crown of Thorns thy Master bore,
The world's great Sovereign, as a Traitor, dy'd.

How was thy Brittania tost!
Forc'd for twelve dismal years t' engage,
With adverse Storms of civil Rage.
A Tempest fell by Furies sent,
So long! so violent!

He

a Kanker Quinsey or Peripn[eumony] . . ." At that time "Quinsey" meant something very different from what it means today. Elsewhere, two good clinical accounts of what was then called "Quinsey" have been quoted[70] and undoubtedly the condition was diphtheritic laryngitis. The significance of "Peripn[eumony]" is not so clear. Laymen often confuse laryngeal obstruction with pneumonia, and besides, pneumonia is a frequent complication of untreated diphtheria. At any rate, there is nothing here in favor of scarlet fever.

It was said that during the Kingston epidemic, "Children while sitting up at play would fall and expire with their playthings in their hands." This is quoted from a source[71] that contains many inaccurate statements and so is of questionable value, but it could hardly have been an imaginary account because it is an accurate, concise, text-book description of a late complication of one of the two diseases—diphtheria.

Sudden heart failure may be seen late in diphtheria. . . . It may occur with few or no premonitory symptoms; as when a child falls dead after walking across a room, or suddenly sitting up in bed, or from some other muscular effort, or possibly as a consequence of passion or excitement. We knew of one little girl who was considered well enough to go coasting and who died suddenly after the effort.[72]

This complication occurs occasionally, but not frequently, in scarlet fever. Douglass does not mention anything comparable to it in his account of the Boston epidemic.

Text-books say that if suitable precautions are not used diphtheria may be carried by physicians and attendants to their own homes, and in this connection there was another difference between the two epidemics. In the "Eastward" towns, multiple deaths in the families of Rev. Ward Clark of Kingston, Dr. Deane of Exeter, Rev. John Brown of Haverhill, Rev. Pain Wingate of Amesbury, Dr. Joseph Hills of Newbury, Rev. Benjamin Allen of Purpoodock, and in the families of many other ministers and physicians is fair evidence that the disease was carried by a third person. In Boston this feature of the epidemic was absent and the selectmen considered it significant enough to advertise the fact:

---

[70] *New York Gazette*, Feb. 17-24, 1735/6. Type 6 of Dickinson's *Observations*. See also, Caulfield, E.: An Essay on the Rattles. J. Pediat., 1936. Feb., p. 226

[71] Farmer and Moore: *Collections, Topographical, Historical and Biographical*, etc. loc. cit.

[72] Holt and Howland: *Diseases of Infancy and Childhood*. 1922, p. 996.

The Practitioners and their Families have not been seized with this Distemper in a more remarkable manner (and as it happened not so much) than other Families in Town, even than those Families who live in solitary Parts thereof.

In the histories of some of the other towns, later to be described, there is additional evidence that two diseases comprised the "throat distemper" epidemic. Not a single item has been found about the New Hampshire epidemic that is not compatible with the diagnosis of diphtheria, yet there is a great deal of evidence that cannot possibly be explained on the assumption that scarlet fever alone was responsible for it all. But before the diagnosis of two separate epidemics can be finally accepted there is one apparent discrepancy to be explained. It will be recalled that the first fatal case (How) during the Boston scarlet fever epidemic had become infected while visiting in Exeter and it was clearly an instance of direct contact. Douglass, who probably saw the patient, relates his history:

> He was lately arrived from Exeter to the Eastward, where his Brother died of this Illness; his Symptoms were great prostration of Strength, a speck in one of his Tonsils, colliquative Sweats, Pulse not high and full, but low, hard, stringy unequal and more frequent than natural, deglutition good to the last, no Sphacelation in the Throat, no eruption; from a rash inconsiderate opinion of forcibly quelling the malignity, he was thrice let blood, had some Emeticks and Catharticks administered, and by profuse evacuations was gradually reduced, so as to die of a gentle decay of natural strength, the 6th Day of Illness.

This boy did not have scarlet fever. He contracted diphtheria in Exeter, returned to live with his mother in Boston and it is probable that very few children were exposed. The house was guarded by a "watch" and "no infection was observed to spread in that Quarter of the Town." In spite of contemporary opinion, the Boston scarlet fever epidemic had no relation to the How case whatsoever; that epidemic was first observed in the opposite end of the town and was well under way before How arrived in Boston.

Why the "throat distemper" was more severe in some Massachusetts towns than in others can be more readily explained on the basis of two separate epidemics, but without detailed records and clinical descriptions it is almost impossible to tell which disease prevailed in any particular town. In Boston, as in New Hampshire, the distemper was not considered to be contagious, so with two large foci of infection and unrestricted travel either disease or both could break out at various times. Undoubtedly there were numerous diphtheria carriers emigrating from the "Eastward," but records like those of the How case are not easily found. Scarlet fever carriers also cannot be easily traced, but in this connection there is an interesting letter in the Massachusetts Historical Society written by the Rev. Hugh Adams of Durham to Nathan Prince of Harvard. It is dated April 22, 1736, which was shortly after the Boston scarlet fever epidemic had reached a peak. Adams was concerned about his son who was supposedly still suffering from the effects of diphtheria

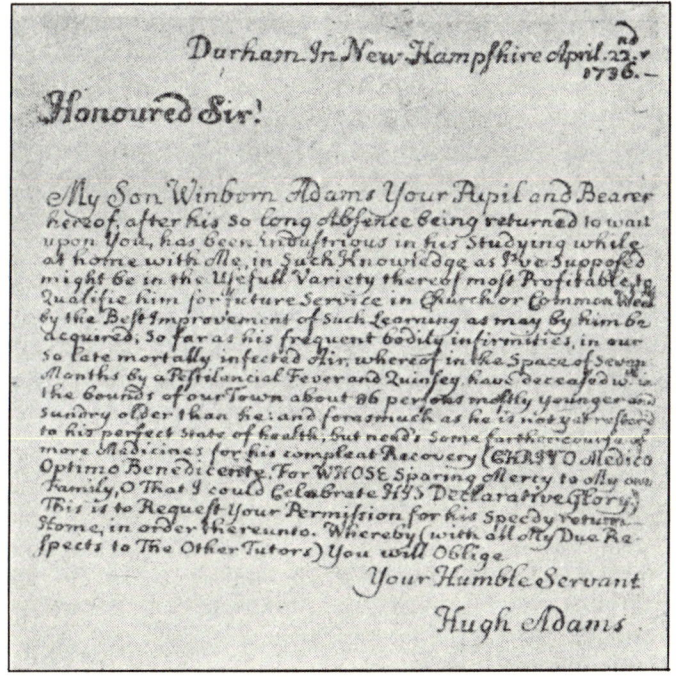

(Courtesy of the Massachusetts Historical Society.)

contracted during the Durham epidemic. The father may not have been alarmed about the rapidly spreading Boston epidemic, nevertheless he wrote:—". . . This is to Request your Permission for his speedy return Home . . ." The son returned to Durham; and it is probable that many others in Boston and vicinity 'speedily returned home' at the height of the epidemic and spread scarlet fever over all New England.

The Boston physicians were very much aware that the "throat distemper" of the country towns was not accompanied by a rash and was more fatal than the Boston kind, yet they became more and more convinced that it was all the same disease and explained the differences in a very clever way. Their theory was that the distemper was caused by some "morbifick matter" in the blood and that it was only necessary to prescribe some efficacious remedies which would allow the poisons to reach the skin surface, evaporate through the pores, and thereby produce a rash. This rash was an indication of successful treatment and offered a plausible explanation of the high mortality in New Hampshire. There the people lived near "salt water damps"; they were "great pork eaters"; and, of course, they never had the proper medical attention. Therefore, the rash was "noticeable only in a few." In Boston, on the other hand, the patients were more vigorous, lived in the pleasant Boston atmosphere, and had excellent physicians who always prescribed effective remedies. Needless to say, the rash invariably appeared and very few were lost. The Boston people had many reasons to be thankful.

This "morbifick matter" theory was not new and had been applied to other diseases many years before, yet it explained the "throat distemper" facts so well that the Boston doctors became thoroughly convinced that it was the only true explanation. More than any other factor, this theory was responsible for the confusion of scarlet fever with diphtheria, and the two diseases were regarded as different manifestations of the same disease for at least another century. Diphtheria came to be known as "canker" and scarlet fever as "canker rash" and it was not until almost very recent times that the two diseases were proved to be distinct. In certain respects, this "morbifick matter" theory has influenced kitchen medicine for generations and persists down to this day. Every grandmother knows that some diseases are more serious "when the rash strikes inward," and this persistent lore is the basis for that well-known treatment for the measles which consists of hermetically sealing up the sick-room, the liberal use of sweaters, woolen blankets, hot baths, and all sorts of warm drinks in order to "bring out a good rash" and thereby rid the body of its poisons.

VI

MASSACHUSETTS

> What mourning Sighs, and loud Out-cries,
> comes from the Eastern Towns
> Of Children crying, and others dying,
> which makes a doleful Sound.
> —A Lamentation.

Most of the old towns between Casco Bay and Boston were connected by a road which ran roughly parallel to the coast and far enough inland to avoid the many small inlets, marsh lands, and sandy dunes. A few weeks after the Kingston outbreak the disease invaded Kittery and Hampton Falls, two important trading centers along this road. From Kittery the infection was carried northward into Maine and from Hampton Falls southward across disputed territory into the Province of Massachusetts Bay. Amesbury[73] and Salisbury[74] were soon involved, and by September the epidemic had crossed the Merrimac River and like an invading army concentrated its forces at Newbury before it started down the old Bay Path towards Boston.

Newbury, which at that time included Newburyport, was only about ten miles south of Hampton Falls and the inhabitants must have heard about the New Hampshire epidemic, though it does not appear that they were aware of any direct relation. They could explain their own distress without reference to any sickness in the neighboring towns. During the previous summer there had been a plague of huge black caterpillars such as had never been seen before, and the leaves on the trees and bushes had been destroyed until the country-side was as barren as in winter. These caterpillars were indeed a nuisance: "No river or pond could stop them. They could swim like dogs, and travel in unaccountable armies and completely cover whole houses and trees. Cart and carriage wheels would be dyed green from the numbers they crushed in progress."

---

[73] *Boston News-Letter*, Oct. 2-9, 1735. D. W. Hoyt: *Old Families of Salisbury and Amesbury*. 1902, ii, 493, mentions numerous baptisms "By Reason of Dangerous Sickness" during August and September 1735. Most of the multiple deaths in the *Amesbury Vital Records*, however, occurred during 1736—see Clough, Currier, Fowler, Lowel, and Winget families.

[74] The only evidence of the distemper in Salisbury, as in a few other Massachusetts towns, is the finding of multiple deaths in the *Vital Records*; see Eaton, Flanders, French, and Hook families.

After an effective Sunday sermon the caterpillars disappeared, but it was thought that the myriads of decomposing carcasses had infected the air and caused the epidemic. There is an anecdote, a little more weird, in the diary of Stephen Jacques:[75]

Thursday, Oct 29th. My wife went into a chamber, that was locked, to fetch candels, that was in a bushel under a bed, and as she kneeled down and took her candels and laid them on the bed and thrust back the half bushel, there came out a child's hand. She saw the fingers, the hand, a streked boy's cote or sleeve, and upon sarch there was no child in the chamber. On Thursday a fortnite after, my Steven's son Henry died. The next Thursday Ebenezer died. The next Monday morning his eldest son Stephen died.

At first, the disease did not cause much concern and it was reported[76] that "there is but six that have died within a Week, and the rest that are sick are likely to recover." That was written in the autumn, but before the winter was over the epidemic spread throughout the town and there were over one hundred deaths between September and the last of December, 1735.[77] Eighty-one children died on Chandler's Lane (Federal Street) alone. Multiple deaths were numerous.[78] The deaths of the eight Boynton children have been mentioned, but when four of them were buried in a single grave, even the New York newspapers noted the event and remarked:—"the like sorrowful Instance seldom known in this part of the world."[79]

Dr. John Fitch (1709-1736), son of the Rev. Jabez Fitch of Portsmouth, was a practising physician in Newbury at this time. After his graduation from Harvard College (1728), he studied under Dr. Nathaniel Sargeant of Hampton and later settled in Newbury where his medical talents and exceptional character were gratefully appreciated. When the sickness first appeared he became intensely interested in its cause and treatment but after a tedious and trying year of practice, he, himself, contracted the disease and died— one of the first American martyrs to science.

---

[75] J. Coffin: *Hist. of Newbury*, p. 204; E. V. Smith: *Hist. of Newburyport*, p. 46.

[76] *Boston News-Letter*, Oct. 9-16, 1735.

[77] *Boston Evening Post*, Jan. 5, 1736.

[78] *Newbury Vital Records*: Bailey, Brown, Chase, Coffin, Dole, Emery, Fowler, Hale, Hodkins, Huse, Kelly, March, Merrill, Mors, Ordway, Pike, Rogers, and Sawyer families.

[79] *New York Gazette*, Jan., 1735/6.

He was happy in a very easy and pleasant natural Temper, polite in his Address, and virtuous in his whole Behaviour, which greatly recommended him to the good Opinion of all who were acquainted with him, and gained him the Affections of those with whom he conversed, so as to be extensively useful, particularly in the practice of Physick.

Tho' in the Distemper which has so long prevailed in these Parts, few Gentlemen of the Faculty had equal none greater success, yet it proved fatal to himself, for after a few Days Sickness in which from the first the Symptoms were violent and threatening, his natural infirm Constitution, yet more debilitated by his late excess in Business, yielded to the Distemper, in the 27th Year of his Age; by whose Death, tho' we trust it was gain to himself, the Publick hath sustained an heavy Loss, and accordingly it is greatly lamented.[80]

Byfield, a parish of about eighty-five families in the southwest part of Newbury, also became involved in the autumn of 1735, and within a year there were over a hundred deaths, which was said to have been more than a seventh of the total population.[81]

For a time it seemed that Rowley, a few miles south of Newbury on the Bay Path, would escape a serious epidemic. There were occasional multiple deaths during the winter of 1735-36, mostly in that part of the town that was close to Byfield, and by spring it was supposed that the distemper had abated throughout the "Eastward." This was only an apparent calm, for on the first day of summer, two-year-old John Plumer, of the second parish, died—"the first child that died in this parish of ye sore sickness of which great numbers have died in Neighbour Parishes"—and for the next six or eight months the epidemic spread with its usual violence.[82] In the second parish, where there had been less than eight deaths annually, forty-six children died, and it has been estimated that in Rowley and neighboring parishes, two hundred, or one-eighth of the total population, died during the first year of the sickness.[83]

---

[80] *Boston Gazette*, Nov. 1-8, 1736; *Boston News-Letter*, Oct. 28-Nov. 4, 1736.
[81] *Boston News-Letter*, Oct. 14-18, 1736; Morse and Parish: *Compendious Hist. of New Engl.*, p. 329.
[82] *Rowley Vital Records*: Multiple deaths in the Adams, Blaisdel, Brocklebank, Chaplin, Cheney, Clark, Cooper, Dickinson, Easty, Gerrish, Goodridge, Harriman, Hazzen, Hidden, Jackman, Johnson, Lunt, Moody, Northend, Noyse, Palmer, Pearson, Perley, Pingree, Russell, Saunders, Steward, Stickney, Tenney, Thurlow, Turner, Wallingford, Wheeler, and Woodman families. More multiple deaths in three branches of the Cressey Family—*New Engl. Hist. & Geneal. Reg.*, April, 1877, 201.
[83] Gage: *Hist. of Rowley*. 1840, pp. 430, 432.

There are no clinical descriptions available, but there is good reason to believe that the disease in Newbury, Byfield, and Rowley was diphtheria, or the same that was present in New Hampshire. The very high death-rate and the frequency of multiple deaths are the two outstanding characteristics that differentiate it from scarlet fever, at least from the type of scarlet fever that was prevalent at that time. In Ipswich, however, the history of the epidemic is somewhat confusing and in the absence of detailed descriptions only a tentative diagnosis can be made. In April 1736, the *Boston News-Letter* reported:

'Tis said, the Distemper is abated at the Eastward; . . . 'Tis also said, that several have lately died of a Scarlet Fever at Ipswich and other Places.

The *Ipswich Vital Records* show that Michael Farley lost five children in April, 1736, four of them in one week, and during the next two years numerous families lost three or four children apiece.[84] The family records of Mark and Hephzibah How, in particular, reveal definite evidence of a malignant contagious disease:

Lucy	died	November	5,	1736
Mary	"	"	15,	"
Aaron	"	"	18,	"
Hannah	"	"	18,	"
Abijah	"	"	21,	"
Mark	"	"	24,	"
Love	"	"	28,	"
Moses	"	"	28,	"

It was said that John Abbott, a neighbor, also lost eight children about the same time and that Nathaniel Cross lost seven during one month in 1738.[85] From a superficial consideration of these brief facts it appears that scarlet fever was the prevailing disease in Ipswich. During 1736, scarlet fever was present in a number of other Massachusetts towns and from the date of the *News-Letter* item (April 15-22, 1736) one may surmise that the Ipswich scarlet fever was a part of the same epidemic that had been present in Boston for the previous six months. But the Ipswich records show

---

[84] *Ipswich Vital Records*: Two or more deaths in the Abbe, Appleton, Baker, Bennet, Boardman, Brown, Burnam, Choate, Fuller, Gibson, Hart, Heard, Jackson, Jewet, Kimball, Knowlton, Lull, Neland, Pierce, Pottar, Safford, Shatchwell, Sherwin, Smith, Treadwell, Trucker, and Webber families.

[85] *Boston News-Letter*, Dec. 2-9, 1736. *New York Gazette*, Feb. 21-28, 1737/8. Felt: *Hist. of Ipswich, Essex, and Hamilton*, p. 338.

many multiple deaths which are difficult to explain unless it is assumed that scarlet fever in Ipswich was a great deal more malignant than in any other town. I believe that the Ipswich records are more satisfactorily explained in another way. While the scarlet fever epidemic was spreading out from Boston the diphtheria epidemic was descending from the north, and in Essex county they travelled along the old Bay Path at the very same time but in opposite directions. It is not necessary to assume that there was only one disease in Ipswich. Indeed, if diphtheria was epidemic in almost every little town to the north of Ipswich, it was probably present in Ipswich too, because the Ipswich epidemic has the same characteristics as the epidemics in the other northern towns. Although scarlet fever may have caused many deaths during 1736, I believe that the Farley, How, Abbott, and Cross children died from diphtheria, the more malignant of the two diseases, or possibly from a combination of the two. That the How children, at least, died of diphtheria is suggested by the town records which state that they died of "cancre quinsy"—an eighteenth century term for laryngeal obstruction.[86]

There is evidence of the distemper at Wenham (1737),[87] Beverly (1736-37),[88] and Salem (1736-37);[89] in the brief facts concerning Marblehead conclusive proof of two separate epidemics can be found. According to the *New York Gazette*, in August, 1737, when the pestilence was at its height in Marblehead, forty-five deaths occurred within fifteen days. "It seems to be a very unaccountable Distemper, no Medicines, which have as yet been apply'd, have any Efficacy to remove, or so much as ease the Patients . . ." This was more than a year after the Boston epidemic and, since Marblehead was only fifteen miles from Boston, some of the physicians, if at all worthy of the name, must have tried the same treatment that had been used in Boston during the previous year with such remarkable success. William Douglass, who went to Marble-

---

[86] D. W. Howe: *Howe Genealogies*. 1929, p. 170.

[87] *New York Gazette*, Feb. 21-28, 1737. *Essex Antiquarian*, vii, 108. Multiple deaths in Batchelder, Dodge, and Patch families. See illustration of the Gott family tombstones. Allen: *Hist. of Wenham*. 1860, p. 127.

[88] *Beverly Vital Records*: Multiple deaths in Conant, Cox, Patch, Smith, Stone, and Trask families. Hall's List of Deaths in Beverly in *Hist. Coll. Essex Inst.*, v, 16. *Boston News-Letter*, Jan. 22-27, 1737.

[89] See illustration of Henchman's Prospectus—the Rev. J. Chipman's report of the north precinct of Salem. *Salem Vital Records*: Judith Pickman.

head to observe the epidemic, still insisted that the high mortality was the result of improper therapy, but in his ingenious explanation he unconsciously solves the mystery and establishes the diagnosis. He said that the first Marblehead epidemic in 1736 was accompanied by "the Eruptive Fever & very few died but their 2d seizure 1737 had no miliary eruption & bad regimen and proved very mortal."[90] In other words, the comparatively mild scarlet fever had spread from Boston to Marblehead on its way up the road to Ipswich in 1736, and the malignant diphtheria epidemic had come down the road from Newbury, Ipswich, and other places and reached a peak in Marblehead during 1737. Douglass' brief description of the Marblehead events cannot be explained by either scarlet fever or diphtheria alone, and so the very man upon whose word many historians rely for a diagnosis of the "throat distemper" was mistaken in his belief that it was caused by one disease.

The infection may have spread to Gloucester, near the tip of Cape Anne, along the road from either Beverly or Ipswich. There is some evidence of the distemper in 1736, but the real epidemic there was in 1738.[91] In a memorial to the General Court, the people of Sandy Bay mentioned that they had lost "thirty-one of their pleasant children by death,"[92] and as there were only twenty-seven families at Sandy Bay, this was probably more than a third of all their children. It is apparent that if the "Scarlet Fever at Ipswich and other Places" was no more severe than that in Boston, it was not an epidemic of scarlet fever at Sandy Bay.

The Gloucester records illustrate another feature of the epidemic, and that is the frequent recurrences of deaths in various branches of certain families. Between March 5 and July 21, 1738, there were four deaths in each of three different branches of the Pool family.[92] In other towns, the Boynton, Cressey, Howe, Lock, and Moulton families had multiple deaths in various branches. William Douglass noted that "in some family constitutions it is generally mortal in others very favourable." But one cannot determine from the records whether this feature should be attributed to family susceptibility, to intimate contact, or to the presence of healthy carriers.

---

[90] *Coll. New York Hist. Soc. for 1918.* N. Y., 1919, p. 196. *Marblehead Vital Records*: Multiple deaths in Norwood, Paramore, Roundey, and Wills families.

[91] *Gloucester Vital Records*: Boynton, Harris, and Pool families.

[92] J. J. Babson: Hist. of Gloucester. 1860, p. 335.

As a general rule, the diphtheria epidemic spread from one town to the next because there was far more communication between neighboring towns than between distant towns, yet there were many exceptions to this rule. Kittery became infected long before its neighboring towns and the disease was also carried directly from Exeter to Boston, although the How case was not the cause of an epidemic. During the spring of 1736, the disease was very prevalent throughout New Hampshire and northeastern Massachusetts, and after this time it is impossible to determine the source of infection for any particular town. Marblehead, for instance, may have received its initial diphtheria infection from Ipswich or Newbury or even from some New Hampshire town. The Massachusetts "throat distemper" was complicated enough by the presence of two separate epidemics, but when it became still more complicated by the unrestricted travel of countless healthy carriers, a detailed explanation of any local epidemic can only be conjectural. Nevertheless, in one or two instances the available records allow some interesting speculation. For example, away off in a little frontier settlement at Dudley, which is fifteen miles south of Worcester, a tragedy occurred in the family of Benjamin and Martha Conant:[93]

Abigail	died	December 29,	1736
John	"	January 5,	1736/7
Benjamin	"	January 6,	1736/7
Asa	"	January 7,	1736/7
Ebenezer	"	January 8,	1736/7

Now there is no other definite evidence of the "throat distemper" in the vicinity of Dudley before 1740-41,[94] and yet these records are so strikingly similar to the records of the "Eastward" towns that there is a temptation to conclude that these children died from diphtheria. If so, how did they get the disease? Dudley was a very small settlement; in fact, Benjamin Conant, the father of these children, was one of the original settlers. There were very few children in the town and certainly no epidemic in 1736, and so it is improbable that these children became infected at church or school or play. There is another and better explanation. Benjamin Conant

---
[93] *Dudley Vital Records.*
[94] Ibid.: Multiple deaths in Bracket, Davis, Howe, Newell, and Thomson families during 1740-41.

originally migrated from Beverly where the "throat distemper" raged during the summer and autumn of 1736, and among the victims were four children of Jonathan Conant, who was related to the Dudley settlers.[95] Therefore, although it is usually hazardous to draw any conclusions from isolated occurrences of multiple deaths, the Dudley episode can be readily explained on the assumption that some member of the Conant family was a diphtheria carrier.

While the diphtheria epidemic was spreading along the Bay Path, another epidemic appeared in Massachusetts directly south of Kingston. There was an old road leading from the Great Pond into Haverhill, about fifteen miles away, and the epidemic may have travelled along this road, though it is also possible that it travelled by way of Amesbury or Newbury and reached Haverhill from the east. This second course may explain the delay, for the Haverhill epidemic did not begin until nearly six months after the Kingston outbreak. At that time, Haverhill consisted of three parishes with a total of about twelve hundred people[96] and, according to the *Vital Records*, which are somewhat incomplete, there had been about ten deaths a year since 1725. The epidemic began in November, 1735, and among the first victims were two of the Whittier children. Although slow in starting, it raged violently for the next two years and Haverhill suffered more than any other Massachusetts town. During 1736 there were 116 deaths, and 130 more during 1737; ninety-eight per cent were under twenty years of age.

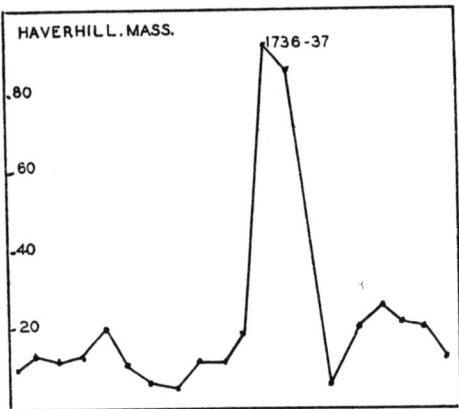

Haverhill, Mass., deaths, 1725-1744. Compiled from vital records published by the Topsfield Historical Society, 1911.

---

[95] *Hist. Coll. Essex Inst.*, v, p. 16; *Hist. and Gen. of the Conant Family*, pp. 180-81.
[96] Estimated.

It was said that nearly every family was afflicted and that more than half of the Haverhill children died.[97] At least sixty families lost two or more children; some of them lost four or five apiece. Twenty-three families were left childless.

The history of these times in Haverhill centers around the Rev. John Brown (1696-1746). He was born in Little Cambridge (Brighton), attended Harvard College (1714), and later married Joanna, a descendant of the celebrated John Cotton. Brown went to Haverhill in 1719 on a salary of "£100, half in corn &c." His epitaph states that he was greatly esteemed for his learning, piety, and prudence, and that his death was justly lamented as a loss to his family, church, and country.[98] During the epidemic, in which he lost three children, he was tireless in his efforts to aid his unfortunate people.

In March, 1737, Daniel Henchman, a Boston bookseller, impressed with the researches of Jabez Fitch in New Hampshire and anxious to gather and publish the Massachusetts figures, sent out a questionnaire to the ministers of various Massachusetts towns. He stated in his prospectus:

> To the Account, when compleated, the Subscriber proposes to annex and publish a pathetick Address, both to Parents and Children, and especially the rising Generation, suitable to such an awful Providence, drawn up by some Reverend Divine, who will please to favour us with a brief Composure, so very seasonable and desireable. And that the Treatise may be more useful, it may be advisable to send Accounts both of the more extraordinary and affecting Instances of the Distemper in particular Persons and Families: As also of the more remarkable Expressions drop'd by the Deceased, especially of the Younger. . . .

It is to be regretted that the statistical part of this contemplated work did not appear, but the plan materialized to some extent, for soon afterwards John Brown published a work that answers the requirements except that the material was confined to the Haverhill epidemic. *A Relation of some Remarkable Deaths among the*

---

[97] Chase: *History of Haverhill.* 1861, p. 306. If "more than half" of the children died, the minimum case fatality was over 50 per cent. Apparently most of the adults were immune. Provided some of the children were immune, the actual case fatality was probably over 70 per cent.

[98] *Coll. Mass. Hist. Soc.*, 2nd Ser., iv, p. 142.

Children of Haverhil under the late Distemper in the Throat with an Address to the Bereaved[99] was printed for Henchman in 1737 and must have been very popular because a second edition, with a

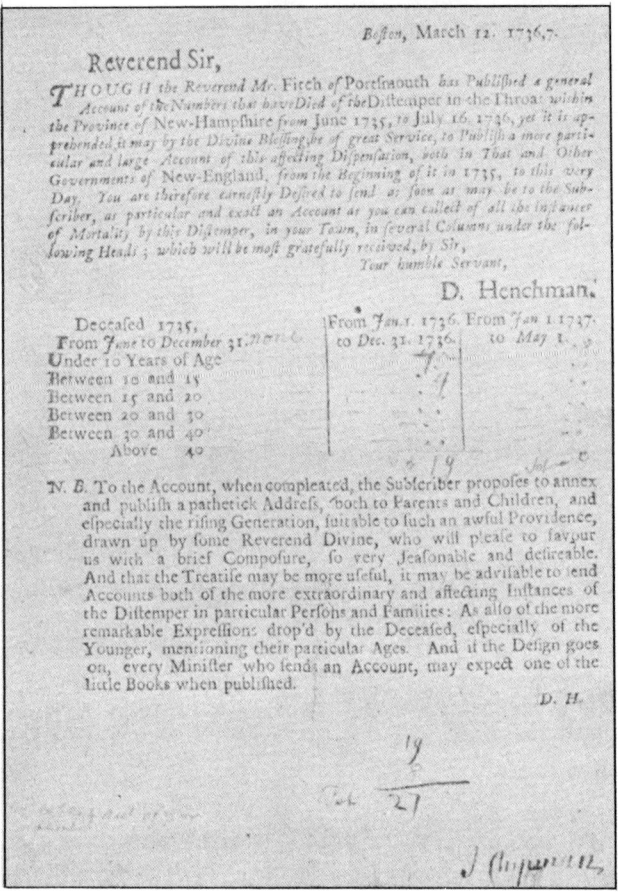

(Courtesy of the Historical Society of Pennsylvania.)

slightly altered title, appeared in 1738 and was advertised for sale "by the dozen." It is a rare, curious, and morbid piece of literature and certainly would not be very popular at the present time, for it

---

[99] Title supplied by Dr. T. F. Capeles of Haverhill, who owns a complete copy of the first edition. Essex Inst. has a second edition. Incomplete editions in Amer. Antiq. Soc. and in Boston Pub. Library.

over-emphasizes the gruesome aspect of contemporary piety, the "remarkable Expressions" being the religious utterances of the feverish, delirious, and exhausted children on the approach of death. Nevertheless, the work is very valuable for in the numerous case histories Brown relates many items of medical interest:

Mrs Betty Bailey, was a loving Companion, Ætat Fifteen, who with her Sister Mrs Molly Bailey, Ætat Thirteen, entered, were a desirable Couple, taken away from the Family of Col. Bailey, Esq. May 5 & 11, 1736, with a Scarlet Fever as well as the throat Distemper . . .

Brown was evidently aware that scarlet fever and "throat Distemper" were entirely separate diseases

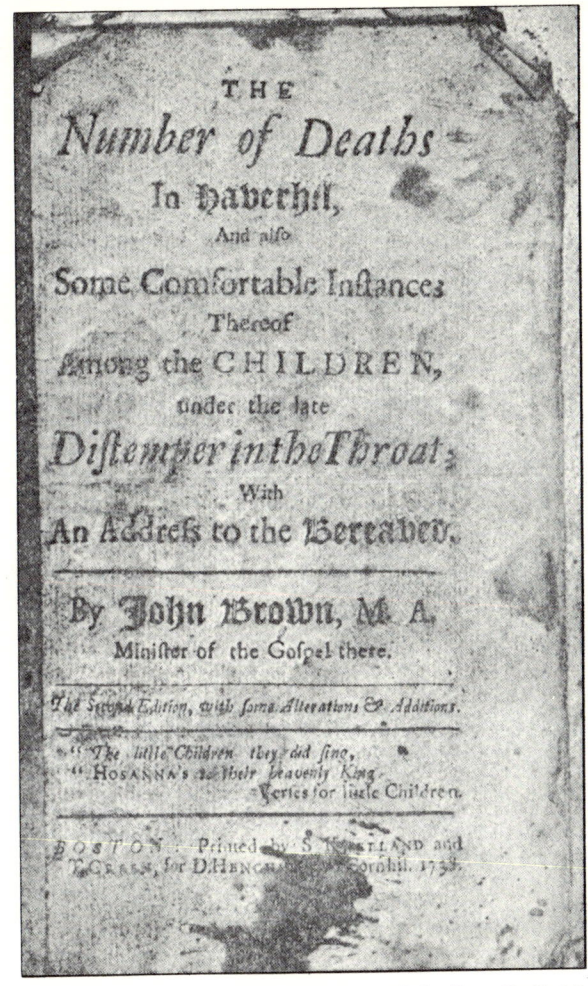

(Courtesy of the Essex Institute)

and as he does not mention scarlet fever in any other case it can be assumed that diphtheria was the prevailing sickness.

Sept 2 1736. Died Susannah Emerson. Aetat Ten. Saturday she complained of Indisposition, and her Mother telling her, She was afraid she was going to be sick, she cried and took on bitterly; but the next Day, when her Mother discovered the Canker in her Throat, she went away as composed as could be, and never said one word. . .

This case was cited as an excellent example of courage in the face of death, but aside from the sentimental aspect, it is the usual story of diphtheria. If the child had had malignant scarlet fever she would have become suddenly sick and a rash would have been immediately evident. That the laity looked for "Canker" in the throat and not for a rash on the body indirectly establishes the diagnosis of the Haverhill epidemic.

Other case histories explain the spread of the disease:

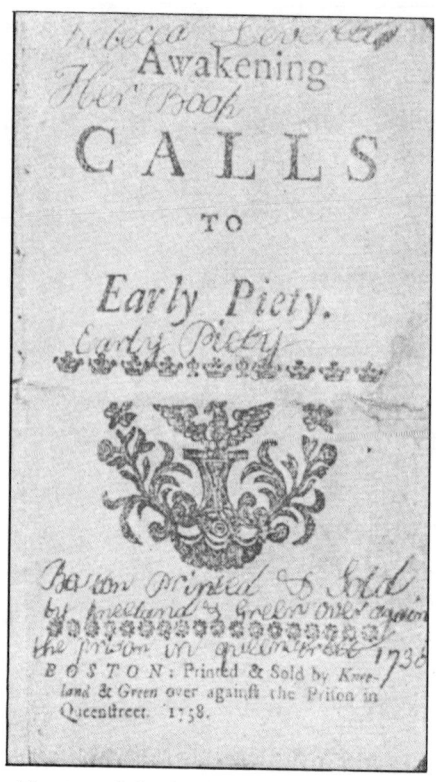
(Courtesy of the American Antiquarian Society.)

> Died Susannah Emerson, Aetat Fifteen. They say she had been a sober little Girl all along, never inclined to be rude or proud as some Girls, but very timerous. Before she was sick, she had been tending a Family of sick Children . . . that all died of the Distemper, and was so much surprised at their Death that sometimes she was almost afraid to go across the Room, but when she her self was seized with *the Canker* exceeding bad, she was no ways distress'd about it, nor ever express'd regret for having been at the House, where in all probability she took the Distemper; . . .

> . . . And one Sabbath-Evening, but two or three Days before he was taken sick, having been to visit a Child of his Sister H———th, that was in a dying State . . .

These are among the few instances throughout the whole epidemic where any idea of contagion was definitely expressed, but Brown relates other instances from which one may conclude that the notions of contagion were very vague:

> Died Susannah Wilson Aetat Seven. After three or four Days Sickness, she gave away her Things to her Elder Sisters, & took the other children in her Arms and kiss'd them . . .

It would have been more "remarkable" if these children had escaped the disease.

The confused history of the Massachusetts epidemic is very well shown by comparing Haverhill with Boston. Both towns were the scenes of great distress during 1736 and to the unsuspecting reader it would seem that the same disease was the cause. But whereas an occasional case of scarlet fever complicated the diphtheria epidemic in Haverhill, in Boston this relation was reversed; Haverhill had abundant instances of multiple deaths in families, Boston few or none; the respective death and fatality rates were strikingly different; and at nearly the same time that about half of the Haverhill children were being carried to their graves, the Boston selectmen were jubilantly proclaiming through the newspapers "that scarce any Distemper, even the most favourable which has at any time prevailed so generally, has produced fewer Deaths."[100]

The *Vital Records* of Bradford,[101] Georgetown,[102] Topsfield,[103] and Wakefield,[104] reveal definite evidence of the distemper in 1736-37. When Andover (1738-39),[105] Middleton (1739),[106] and Lynn (1740),[107] became involved, the epidemic had covered practically all of Essex County, and fourteen hundred children had lost their lives.[108]

In 1738, when the epidemic was still raging in Maine and throughout Essex County, Massachusetts, with no indication of its letting up either in virulence or progress, a timely pamphlet of gruesome verse appeared. The author is unknown. Evans[109] attributes it to Hull Abbott (1702-1774), a minister at Charlestown, but this is undoubtedly an error for the initials "N. N." are found

---

[100] *Boston News-Letter*, Apr. 22-29, 1736.

[101] *Bradford Vital Records*. Multiple deaths in Carlton, Hardy, Jewet, Pearl, Sessions, Tenney, and Wood families.

[102] *Essex Antiquarian*, viii, p. 49. Multiple deaths in Blasdel, Brocklebank, Cooper, and Harriman families.

[103] *Deaths in Topsfield, Essex Inst. Hist. Coll.*, xxxviii, p. 129. Multiple deaths in Peabody, Perkins, Porter, Reddington, and Towne families.

[104] *Wakefield Vital Records*. Multiple deaths in Batt, Burnap, Damon, Parker, Stow, Swayn, and Wiley families.

[105] *Andover Vital Records*. Multiple deaths in Astin, Ballard, Blanchard, Carlton, Clark, Dane, Farrington, Foster, Fice, Lovejoy, Marble, and Peters families.

[106] *Middleton Vital Records*. Multiple deaths in How, Robinson, and Thomas families.

[107] *Zaccheus Collins Diary*. Ms. in Essex Inst.; Lewis and Newhall: *Hist. of Lynn*, p. 325.

[108] *Essex Antiquarian*, 1897, i, p. 10.

[109] *Bibliography of American Literature*. No. 4214. The similarity in meter and theme of this poem to *A Lamentation* suggests the same authorship.

on the last page. Its dismal and melancholy theme continues for seventeen pages, but only a few verses are needed for illustration:

AWAKENING CALLS TO EARLY PIETY

The glorious God, hath cast abroad
   his Anger on this Nation,
And dreadful Wrath, he kindled hath,
   against this Generation.

* * *

Your Souls affair, Children take care,
   you don't procrastinate;
O now begin, to turn from sin,
   before it be too late.

* * *

O may this Call, awaken all
   you Children to amend,
Your sinful Lives: O now be wise
   and mind your latter end.

* * *

O sad Estate, yea Desperate
   will your Condition be,
If you should be found in that day,
   with God at enmity.

So soon as Death, hath stopt your Breath,
   your Soul's must then appear
Before the Judge of quick and dead,
   the Sentence there to hear.

From thence away, without delay,
   you must be Doom'd unto,
A dreadful Hell, where Devils dwell,
   in Everlasting woe.

Where dreadful horrors, amazing terrors,
   shall you encompass round,
Eternally, there you must ly,
   in chains of darkness bound.

I' th' sulph'rous Lake, where direful flakes,
   of Fire doth spread abroad,
Eternally, there kindled by,
   the great Eternal God.

Although the "throat distemper" involved many towns outside of Essex County, only the records of a few of those towns are of particular interest. During the summer and autumn of 1738 there was a decided increase in deaths among the children of Malden, most of them in the Howard, Green, Paine, Sargant, and Upham families.[110] Samuel and Mary (Grover) Upham lost

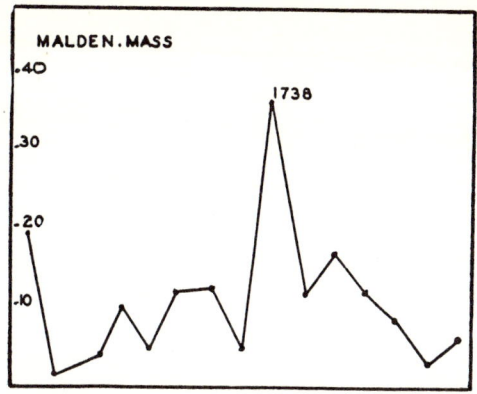

Malden, Mass., deaths, 1730-1744. Compiled from records in the *New Engl. Hist. & Geneal. Reg.*, xii, 242; xiii, 70.

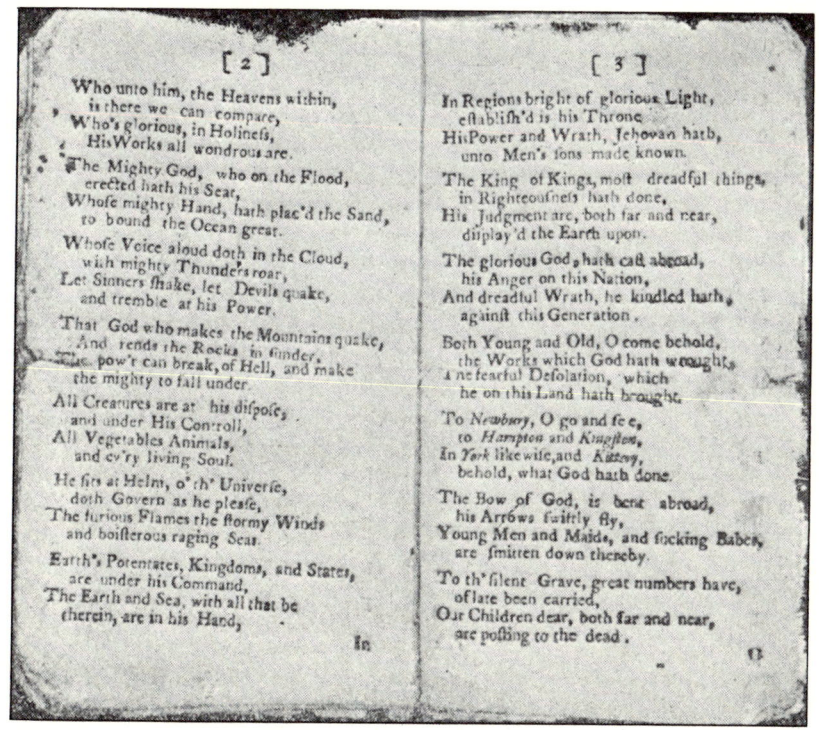

(Courtesy of the American Antiquarian Society.)

Pages from AWAKENING CALLS TO EARLY PIETY

---

[110] *New Engl. Hist. & Geneal. Reg.*, xii, 242; xiii, 70. Corey: *Hist. of Malden*, p. 639.

four, and on the occasion of the "joyful and triumphant Death" of Abigail, the Rev. Joseph Emerson preached his sermon on *Early Piety Encouraged*. Copies of this, and of a second sermon, are now very rare, but only a few lines in one of them have any medical importance:

Moreover, I must take the Freedom to exhort you also, to be helpful to your sick and afflicted Neighbours, as there may be Occasion. Let me tell you, it is an inordinate and sinful Fear that you have of the Distemper, if it keep you from going *nigh* your Neighbours, to tend up them, to *watch* with them, or in any other *Respect* to be helpful to them . . .

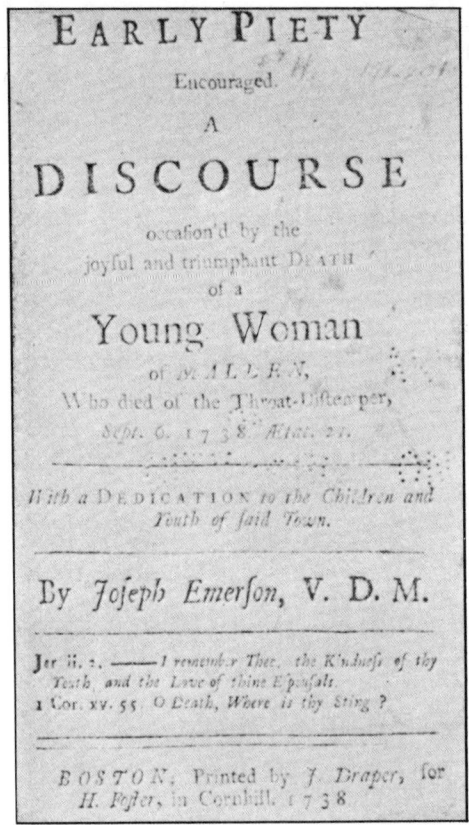

(Courtesy of the Boston Public Library.)

No doubt many Malden people thought that the disease was contagious. William Douglass went to Malden at the time of the epidemic and the diagnosis rests upon his account.[111] He found "no milliary Eruptions but a slow putrid fever" and ulcers in the throat. Douglass was aware that the Malden sickness had a different appearance from the Boston sickness of 1736, so it is more than probable that diphtheria was the cause of the Malden epidemic.

A note in the diary of the Rev. Samuel Dexter of Dedham[112] varies from the usual story concerning most of the Massachusetts towns:

May 26th 1736. This day, a Sovereign, Righteous & Holy God took from us our fifth Son, William, a very Desireable Child, by y^t Awfull Malady wch prevails in ye Country, & Another of my Children, vizt, Ebenezer, lay at

---

[111] *Coll. New York Hist. Soc. for 1918.* 1919, p. 196.
[112] *New Engl. Hist. & Geneal. Reg.*, 1860, xiv, 204.

y̆ᵉ point of Death, wᵐ Gᵈ graciously spar'd & Recover'd, & afterwards, I my self was Visited with it, & yᵉ most, if not all yᵉ family, tho' in moderation.

On account of the date, the proximity of Dedham to Boston, and the "moderation" of the disease, scarlet fever is the probable diagnosis.

There is not sufficient material to warrant separate descriptions, but there is evidence of the distemper in Braintree (1738-39),[113] Brookfield (1738),[114] Eastham (1736),[115] Grafton (1740),[116] Harvard (1739),[117] Lancaster (1740),[118] Lexington (1740),[119] Littleton (1740),[120] Lunenburg (1740),[121] Marlborough (1740),[122] Martha's Vineyard (1740),[123] Milton (1738),[124] Nantucket (1736),[125] Oxford (1740-41),[126] Reading (1736-37),[127] Sherborn (1736),[128] Shrewsborough (1740),[129] Southborough (1740),[130] Sutton (1740-41),[131] Uxbridge (1740-41),[132] Watertown (1737),[133] Westborough (1740),[129] Weston (1736 and 1739-40),[134] and Woburn (1738).[135] Some towns, Medford and Danvers for example, within the path of the epidemic seem to have escaped. I have found no evidence of the epidemic to the west of Worcester county.

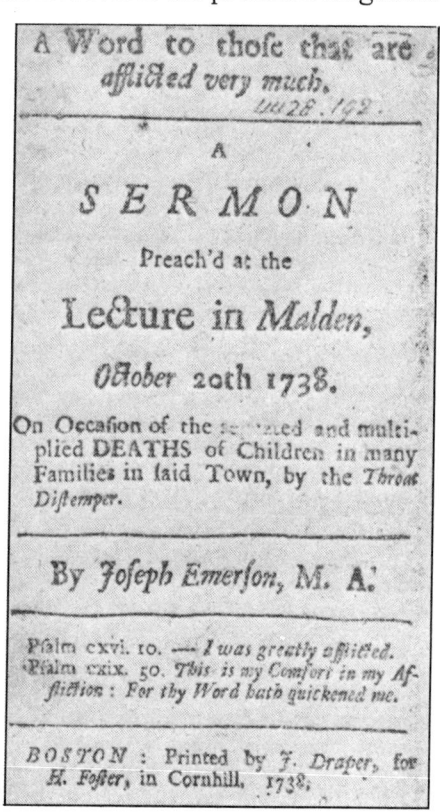

(Courtesy of the Boston Public Library.)

---

[113] *New York Gazette*, Feb. 21-28, 1737/38. *Records of Town of Braintree* (1888): Samuel Pain lost five children in 1739.

[114] *Brookfield Vital Records*. Multiple deaths in Ashely, Gooddel, Goss, Heywood, and Hinds families.

[115] *New England Weekly Journal*, Nov. 2, 1736.

[116] *Grafton Vital Records*. Multiple deaths in Benjamin, Drury, Grover, Merriam, Pratt, and Smith families.

[117] Nourse: *Hist. of Harvard*, 1894, p. 515. Whitcomb and Witherbee families.

VII

A RELAPSE

> And now again I send
> mine Angel through the Land,
> To visit you with sicknesses,
> Which you cannot withstand.
>
> —Earnest Expostulation.

The Boston scarlet fever epidemic quieted down near the end of 1736. During the next few years, William Douglass found

---

[118] H. S. Nourse: *Birth, Marriage and Death Reg. of Lancaster*, p. 158. Moor and Snow families.

[119] *New Eng. Hist. & Geneal. Reg.*, 1858, xii, 267.

[120] *New England Weekly Journal*, July 29, 1740. "Eliz. only child of Samuel Dummer."

[121] *Lunenburg Vital Records*. Carlile and Heywood families.

[122] *Marlborough Vital Records*. Brigham, Stewart, and Taintor families. (See Shrewsborough.)

[123] C. E. Banks: *New Engl. Hist. & Geneal. Reg.*, April, 1896, p. 165.

[124] *Milton Records*, 1900, pp. 217, 220. Davenport and Fenno families. *Journal of Rev. Thomas Smith*, June 27, 1738.

[125] *Boston News-Letter*, June 24-July 1, 1736.

[126] *Oxford Vital Records*. Multiple deaths in Hudson (7 children died within 19 days) and Town families.

[127] Eaton: *Geneal. Hist. of Reading*, 1874, p. 148. *Reading Vital Records*. Multiple deaths in Batt, Burnap, Damon, Emerson, Nickolls, Parker, Stow, Swain, and Townsend families.

[128] *Boston News-Letter*, Feb. 5-12, 1736. *Sherborn Vital Records*. Multiple deaths in Greenwood, Lealand, Sanger, and Warfield families.

[129] "We have an Account that the Throat Distemper has lately proved very mortal in several Towns in the County of Worcester. The Rev. Mr. Cushing of Shrewsborough has bury'd three Children of it, two in a Coffin; Capt Hapgood an hopeful Son of 14 or 15 Years; Mr. Simon Goddard two, and another very bad. In Southborough Lieut. Brigham has bury'd three, and his Brother Thomas (of Marlborough) two. Mr. Beal two; and Mr. Ephraim Ward's wife three Children; and several others have dy'd there. And in Westborough Mr. Hayward two Children, and several others are Sick; and it now begins to come upon them more terribly."—*New Engl. Weekly Journal*, Aug. 12, 1740.

[130] *Southborough Vital Records*. Beals, Brigham, and Britten families. See also Shrewsborough, and *Town of Weston, Births, Marriages and Deaths*, p. 434.

[131] Benedict and Tracy: *Hist. of Sutton*, p. 59.

[132] *Uxbridge Vital Records*. Multiple deaths in Holbrook, Keith, and Rawson families.

[133] *Watertown Records*, Vol. iii, p. 112. Parce family lost four children.

[134] *Boston News-Letter*, Dec. 18-23, 1736; *New Engl. Weekly Journal*, Nov. 13, 1739; *Town of Weston, Births, Deaths and Marriages*, 434 et seq.

[135] *Thomas Smith's Journal*, June 27, 1738. *Woburn Vital Records*. Richardson family lost four.

time for relaxation and amused himself with his economic theories and his maps, while Zabdiel Boylston undoubtedly enjoyed his spacious new home and gardens in the country.[136] When Daniel Henchman sent out his questionnaire in 1737, he, too, believed that the epidemic had definitely passed. There was less anxiety at the selectmen's meetings as they seriously debated about sewers and schools and liquor-permits and the bulls that were grazing on the Common. The storm was over and it appears from the records that, in comparison with other towns, Boston had been more scared than hurt.

Meanwhile, the diphtheria epidemic was slowly descending from the north and had reached Marblehead in 1737 and Malden in 1738, and the Boston people had more reason to be grateful for their superior medical attention and the "laudable and salutary rash" as they frequently read in their newspapers about the frightful devastation in the country towns. In 1739, however, the destructive "Angel" was again seen hovering over the town, and for the benefit of those who had fallen from the state of grace a warning appeared in the form of broadside verse:

> Earnest EXPOSTULATION
>
> O Earth Earth Earth attend,
>   The mighty God hath spoke
> Why will you still offend 'gainst me?
>   Why will you me provoke?
>
> * * *
>
> But O ungrateful Sons,
>   what are you now a doing
> Forsaking of your Father's God
>   and seeking your own Ruin.
>
> * * *
>
> Your tender Children dear,
>   on them mine Hand I've laid,
> But wherefore doth the Lord contend?
>   who hath the Inquiry made?

---

[136] Then called Muddy River, now Boylston St. in Brookline, where his house, built in 1736, still stands.

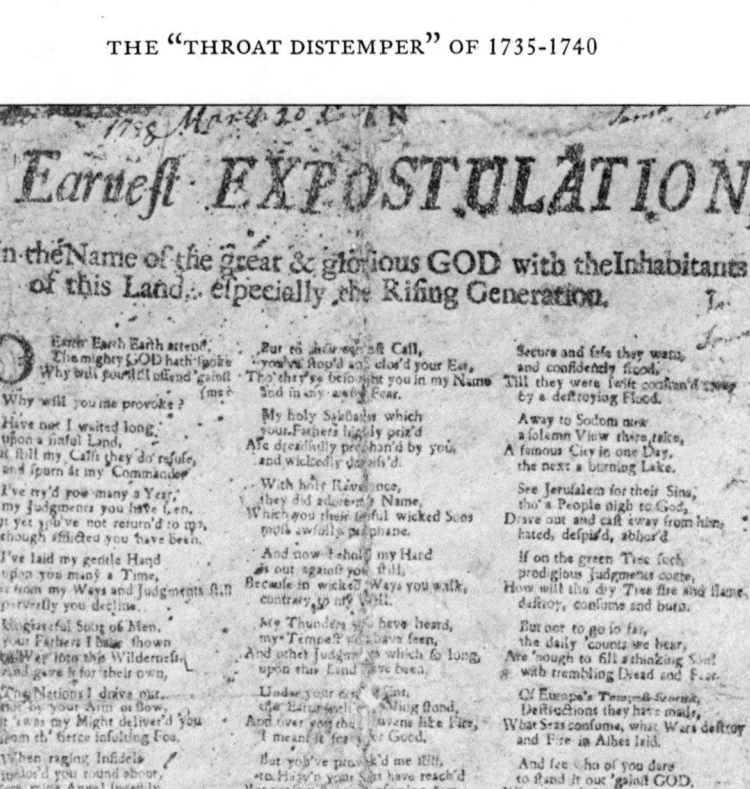

(Courtesy of the American Antiquarian Society. Previously reprinted in *American Broadside Verse*, by O. E. Winslow, Yale University Press, 1930, p. 180.)

> Distressing Judgments still
>   may fast upon you come
> Till in his hot and fiery Wrath,
>   he utterly consume.
>
> * * *
>
> Of all your fine Possessions
>   which he to you hath given,
> And leave you not a Name nor Son
>   under the Copes of Heaven.

It was "earnestly desired that Parents would teach these Lines to their Children!"

There was another increase in deaths in Boston during 1740, but this may have been the normal variation and would be without significance except that there was a similar slight increase in the Dorchester deaths at the same time. All in all, however, there is no evidence of any great amount of sickness in Boston itself, but across the river at Harvard College and surrounding Cambridge there was a definite epidemic. In the preface to a medical book dated at Cambridge in 1740, the printer stated: ". . . now that we have a fresh Alarm by a Return of that astonishing Distemper among us . . ."[137] Three children of one Stedman family and two of another died during the week of June 23rd and about the same time Ruth and Andrew Bordman, grandchildren of the college steward, died.[138] Edward Holyoke, President of Harvard, lost his wife and two-year-old son, William. It was greatly feared that the disease would spread among the students, so it was "therefore Voted, that they be immediately dismissed from the College, and that the vacation begin from this time; and that the Commencement for this year be not until the expiration of the vacation." Holyoke recorded in his diary that a private fast was held at Cambridge on July 2, and the next day,—"The Com[mence]ment put by on account of the throat distemper."[139]

It seems that by a "return" of the epidemic was meant a true recurrence of the previous scarlet fever, but the frequency of multiple deaths suggests diphtheria instead. Additional evidence that diphtheria was present is to be found in *An Account of the Throat Distemper, in a letter from Wm. Douglas M.D. to* ——— *of New*

---

[137] Jonathan Dickinson: *Observations, etc.* Apparently, Cambridge was involved in the scarlet fever epidemic of 1735-36.
[138] L. R. Page: *Hist. of Cambridge*, p. 132.
[139] *Holyoke Diaries, 1709-1856.* Salem, 1911.

York. This publication, said to have been printed by Zenger in 1740, is extremely rare and no copy is available at this time, but undoubtedly it is the same as the letter that Douglass sent in Nov. 1739 to Cadwallader Colden, the physician, scientist, statesman, and philosopher of New York. Douglass frequently wrote to Colden and in this particular letter gave permission for publication.[140]

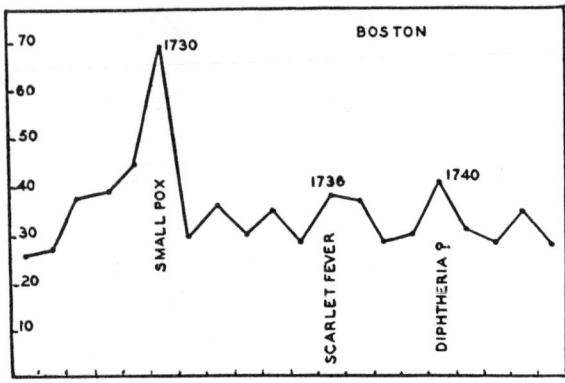

Boston, Mass., deaths per 1000 population, for the period 1725 to 1744. Compiled from statistics in *Census of Boston for the Year 1845*, by Lemuel Shattuck. Boston, 1846.

Although he still believed that he was dealing with the same disease, Douglass' descriptions in 1739 differed in many ways from those of 1736. For example, he said in 1736 that he had observed no instances where the same person was infected twice and that those physicians who had observed second attacks were probably mistaken. At that time, Douglass was right because scarlet fever seldom attacks again the same person within a short period of time. In 1739, however, he admitted that he had seen "Some Second Seizures but with some variation in the symptoms." If Douglass confused the two diseases his statement can be readily understood, particularly when the "variation in the symptoms" points to another disease. He also stated in 1739 that the cases were not accompanied by nausea, that there were ulcers on the skin and mucous membranes, and that the "Tonsils and other parts of the Fauces [were] infiltrated and Speck'd, throwing up from time to time thick cream coloured sloughs (in those who were very bad, from parts further than the Eye can reach) . . ." His most significant statement concerns the respiratory system. Though, in 1736, he mentioned a few cases with laryngeal involvement, a very noticeable feature of his 1739 account was that: "The last complaint is of an oppression and stricture in the upper part of the chest . . . asthmatick breath-

---

[140] *Coll. New York Hist. Soc. for 1918,* 1919, p. 196; 1923, p. 337.

ings, a deep pulmonary hollow hoarse cough, ending in a loud strangled countenance & death."

It is apparent that Douglass had seen the fatal, membranous, diphtheritic croup and, although it is not so apparent whether he had seen those cases in Boston, Marblehead, or Malden, the essential fact remains that in 1739, "throat distemper" to Douglass, at least, and probably to many others, included cases of diphtheria. Therefore, the so-called "return" to Boston and Cambridge was not necessarily a true recurrence of the previous scarlet fever. More probably it was the "throat distemper" in its other form. "Returns" also occurred in other towns and further complicate the history of the Massachusetts epidemic. Sometimes they were spurious "returns"—unrelated to the previous infection—and sometimes the epidemics did actually recur, especially in those towns where diphtheria caused the initial outbreak.[141]

It is difficult to trace the "throat distemper" in Massachusetts after 1740. A proclamation in 1741, which mentions "that awful Distemper whereby so many of the children of this people have been cut off . . ." and the *Vital Records* of many of the smaller towns show that it had by no means disappeared, but there are fewer contemporary comments probably because it was no longer "new." From the meager records, particularly after measles[142] and influenza[143] had appeared, it is almost impossible to make a satisfactory diagnosis. Besides, there were other important events to divert the people's attention. The "War of Jenkins' Ear" had been declared in 1739, and soon after, Whitefield and Tennant came preaching new religious doctrines. Then Jonathan Edwards, in the Connecticut River Valley, had caught his second wind and his voice echoed over the hills to the Atlantic shores. Indeed, the very

---

[141] See Hampton graph.

[142] *New Engl. Hist. & Geneal. Reg.*, 1881, xxxv, 28. *Diary of Paul Dudley*, Roxbury, 1740. He writes: "Jan. 8. Measles continue in many Towns . . . Feb. 5. Measles prevail in many towns and the throat distemper yet in the Land. . . April 9 . . . The Rash pretty brief [mild?]—and so the Measles. . . June. The Throat Distemper got to Cambridge. Several died particularly Madam Holyoke. . . Nov. The Throat distemper in many parts of the Province and very mortal." Dudley apparently distinguished the "Rash" (scarlet fever?) from measles and "Throat Distemper" (diphtheria).

[143] *New York Gazette*, Feb. 21-28, 1737/8; Benedict and Tracy: *Hist. of Sutton*, 1878, p. 59.

devil himself was preparing for his leap from the steeple of the Ipswich church, for the "Great Awakening" was now definitely under way and the "throat distemper" with everything else was crowded off the stage.

VIII

CONNECTICUT

> And now behold my Hand
> is out against you still,
> Because in wicked Ways you walk,
> contrary to my Will.
> —Earnest EXPOSTULATION.

Little is known about the "throat distemper" in Connecticut,[144] chiefly because contemporary writers, more impressed by the startling events in the other provinces, seldom mentioned Connecticut in their accounts. It was taken for granted that the Connecticut epidemic was a part of the "Eastern Distemper" and there was no contemporary student, such as Jabez Fitch in New Hampshire or William Douglass in Boston, interested enough to study the disease. It has seemed worth while, nevertheless, to gather together the few and disconnected reports, not only because they have never before been assembled but also because they are of considerable epidemiologic importance when considered with other phases of the epidemic. A review of the facts in their chronological sequence reveals a number of interesting features concerning geographical progress, mortality, and diagnosis.

The Connecticut epidemic began, not in the regions close to Massachusetts, as one might reasonably expect, but in Stamford in the southwest corner of the colony. Although two children of Caleb Smith died within a few days of each other during the autumn of 1735, the multiple deaths in the family of Joseph and Mary Smith are the first certain evidence of an epidemic:

John	died	January	9	1735/6
Sarah	"	"	9	"
Hannah	"	"	17	"
Abigail	"	"	18	"
Isaac	"	"	25	"

---

[144] Unless otherwise specified, the material for this chapter was taken from manuscript copies of town records in the Conn. State Library at Hartford. When "son," "daughter," or "child" was mentioned, I have assumed the age to be under twenty years.

The town records do not give the cause of death, but about a month later the *Boston News-Letter* (Feb. 19-26, 1736) reported:

> We have an Account from Connecticut, That the Distemper that has for some Months past prevail'd at the Eastward, has now got into the Western Part of that Colony, where several Children and Young People have lately died; particularly at Stamford, where one Mr. John [sic] Smith has buried Five Children in a little more than a Fortnight; and some Families in that Town that had but Three or Four Children have buried them all.

The severity of the Stamford epidemic cannot be learned from the town records because they are noticeably incomplete in not even mentioning the other families that lost "Three or Four Children," but the records do mention other multiple deaths later in 1736. The *News-Letter* identifies the disease as "throat distemper" but, as has been pointed out, that could mean either scarlet fever or diphtheria. During the epidemic, Nathaniel Hubbard, a Stamford physician, wrote to Henry Lloyd of Lloyd's Neck across the Sound[145] and suspecting that some of the Lloyd children were suffering from the disease, he advised:

> ... You may know this Distemper by the following Symptoms Viz: A hot pricking pain about the throat and Ears, white specks in the Throat, At first a white Tongue then yellow & if the fever be great it grows black, some time a swelling under the Throat, if the Fever be very high restlessness, watery Eyes, Paleness of the Face, with external coldness & great dr[ought] In which Case give Saffron tea or something to drive the fever out. My hearty respects at home. I am Sir
>
> Your obliged & Dutiful Kinsman.

From Hubbard's failure to mention any rash, together with the frequent multiple deaths, one may be fairly certain that diphtheria was the cause of the Stamford epidemic.

Not much can be said about the other shore towns of Fairfield County,[146] chiefly because of incomplete records, but in New Haven there was a definite epidemic with an unusual variation. Timothy Dwight,[147] writing in 1811, said: "About the year 1736 the Angina Maligna was prevalent and extensively fatal." The source

---

[145] *Coll. New York Hist. Soc.*, 1927. *Papers of the Lloyd Family.* i, 349.
[146] There is slight evidence of an epidemic about 1738.
[147] Timothy Dwight: *Statistical Account of New Haven*, p. 63.

of Dwight's information has not been ascertained, but other slight evidence that the epidemic began in 1736 is to be found on tombstones in the Grove Street Cemetery.[148] As the names of many children who died during 1736-1739 are not mentioned in the town records,[149] the graph constructed upon those records does not show the full extent of the epidemic. As in one or two other Connecticut towns it probably smouldered a while before bursting into full flame. The statistics, though incomplete, reveal that the peak was reached in 1739 and this is confirmed from other sources:

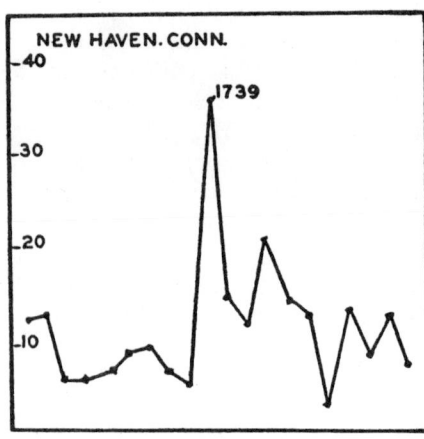

New Haven, Conn., deaths, 1730-1749.

We hear from Connecticut That the Throat Distemper rages very much at New Haven, and that one Mr. [Samuel] Mix of that Place, who had five children, and buried them all in a little more than a Week's time.[150]

The Rev. Daniel Wadsworth mentions in his diary:[151]

July 28 1739. This day heard yt Samuel only son of Mr Daniel Edwards of New Haven died on thursday of ye throat distemper. Aug 14 1739. This day set out on a Journey for my health in Com-

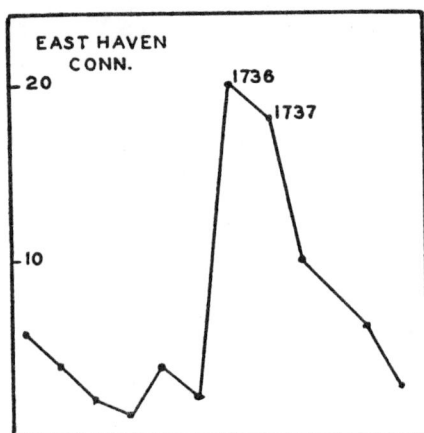

East Haven, Conn., deaths, 1730-1741.

---

[148] F. B. Dexter: *New Haven Tombstone Inscriptions*, in *New Haven Hist. Soc. Coll.*, iii.

[149] Multiple deaths in the families of Samuel Barns, Samuel Bishop Jr., Abner Bradley, John Bradley Jr., Ezekiel Sanford, and the Rev. Mr. Joseph Noyes. *Vital Records of New Haven*, 1917.

[150] *Boston News-Letter*, August 23-30, 1739.

[151] *Diary of the Rev. Daniel Wadsworth.* Hartford, 1894, p. 40.

pany with M^r. Colton, travelled as far as New Haven, the throat distemper prevails there.

The epidemic was complicated by the prevalence of influenza in 1737 and of measles in 1739 (Dwight). There are no detailed case descriptions at hand so the diagnosis of "throat distemper" must suffice.

The summer of 1736 was unusually hot and dry, and during the last half of the year the epidemic raged violently along the Connecticut shore. In East Haven, then a parish of New Haven, it was very severe, and in a population of about two hundred people there were twenty-six deaths under twenty years of age. It began in the autumn and continued throughout the winter.[152]

From 1730 to 1735 there were about three deaths annually among the children of Guilford, which at that time included East Guilford (now Madison). During the autumn of 1736, thirty-eight children died.[153] A sermon by the Rev. Jonathan Todd[154] throws some light upon the nature of the disease:

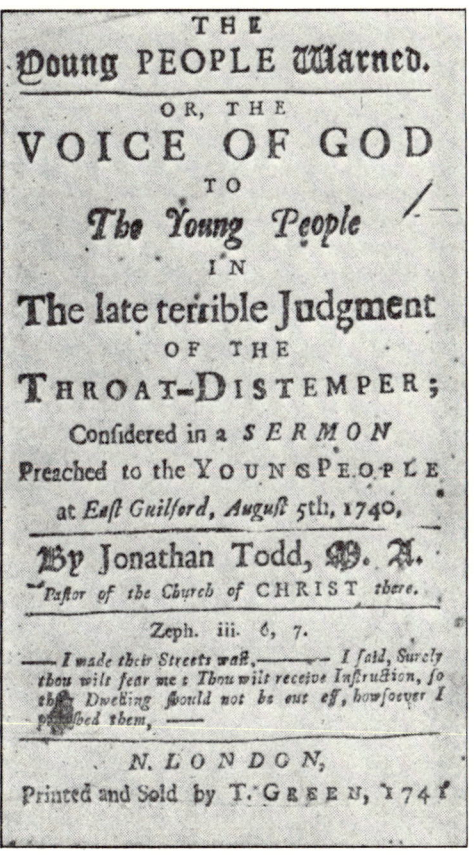

(Courtesy of the Connecticut Historical Society.)

He must be a Stranger indeed in these Parts of the World, who hath not heard of the Desolations made in Sundry Parts of the Country, by that Distemper, that is usually called, The Throat-Distemper.

---

[152] Stephen Dodd: *East Haven Register*, 1910, p. 40.
[153] Samuel Fitch, Ebenezer Parmele, Stephen Spencer, and Capt. Timothy Stone lost two or more children apiece.
[154] Jonathan Todd: *The Young People Warned*. . . . N. London, 1741.

Near Five years ago [the sermon was printed in 1741] we in this Parish were Visited with the same; and sundry very pleasant and hopeful Young Persons were taken away. Since which Time, we have had an Account of more awful Desolations made by it, in many other Places.

Near the Latter End of July last, a very hopeful, serious and likely Young Person, named Prudence Bishop, the Eldest Daughter of Mr. John Bishop, was taken Sick amongst us; At first indeed, we hoped, that her Sickness might be only a hard Cold, a common sore throat attended with a Feaver, or the Effects of a Rash, as we called a Distemper, that was then among us.

But her Sickness presently increased, and she was brought into uncommon Difficulty and Distress. The justly Famous and well known Physician of these Parts was consulted; who judged her Sickness to be the Throat-Distemper. And to be short, the Distemper made Quick Work and carried her off, August 2d, and her Corps was interred on Lords-Day, August 3d.

My interpretation of these statements is that scarlet fever was present in East Guilford in 1740 and that the laity had not detected any similarity between this "Rash" and the disease that had caused the 1736 epidemic; in other words, although both diseases were accompanied by sore throat, the 1736 disease was not accompanied by a rash and therefore was diphtheria. Throughout the history of the "Distemper," the laity seldom confused the two diseases. The "justly Famous and well known Physician," who was either Jared Eliot or Dr. Gale, was undoubtedly familiar with the prevailing medical theories and probably believed that Prudence Bishop had the 1736 disease but in a different form. On the other hand, it is possible that she did not have a rash and that she actually had the 1736 disease; perhaps she had both scarlet fever and diphtheria. At any rate, regardless of the Bishop case, it seems to me that if the "throat distemper" of 1736 had been accompanied by a rash, the Guilford people would have been more alarmed by the "Rash" that was present in 1740. Now, if it is true that diphtheria was present in 1736 and scarlet fever in

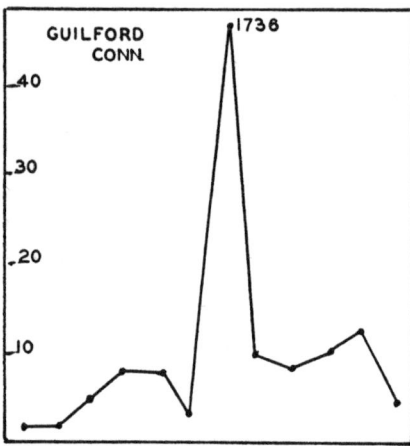

Guilford, Conn., deaths, 1730-1741.

1740, it is interesting to compare the effects of the two diseases upon the same community. In 1740, the increase in deaths was very slight and there are no instances of multiple deaths to be found that year.

Continuing eastward along the shore, we find that in Saybrook, as in New Haven, the epidemic smouldered for a while before it reached a peak in 1739. Twenty-five of the thirty-one deaths (80 per cent) were among children under twenty years of age.[155] In Old Lyme, across the river from Saybrook, two sons of John Denison and two daughters of Benjamin DeWolf died in 1736. The Old Lyme records are not subject to statistical analysis.

The diary of Joshua Hempstead,[156] grandson of one of the first settlers of New London, gives an intimate account of colonial life, and the following extracts were written at the time of the New London epidemic:

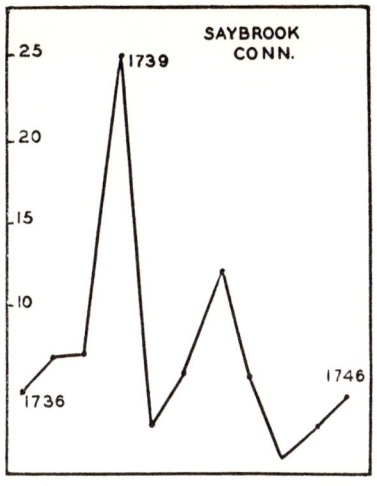

Saybrook, Conn., deaths among children, 1736-1746.

1736, May Thursd 27 I was at home al day Diging Stones &c. A Child 6 or yeare old of Thos Hawkins was buried yesterday with the Distemper in the throat. Several of his Children are Sick with it & Wife & Some others. . . June Thurd.3 fair. I was about home foren. aftern I went over the ferry went to Stonington on my young hipt mare Robert & his wife on Pierponts

---

[155] The Saybrook Church Records (Ms. copy in Conn. Hist. Soc.) show the cumulative effect of the epidemic:

Nathaniel Parker	lost two	children in	1736
Jedidiah Dudley	" three	"	" 1737
Deacon Blague	" "	"	" "
John Whittlesey	" two	"	" 1739
Samuel Clark	" four	"	" "
Richard Dickinson	" "	"	" "
Zebulon Dudley	" "	"	" "
Isaac Jones	" two	"	" "
Samuel Willard	" "	"	" "

[156] *Diary of Joshua Hempstead of New London.* New London County Hist. Soc., 1901.

Horse Benja Hempsted & my Nattee on the black mare & my Grandaughter Abigail behind me wee got there by daylight to Son Minors he is gone to Boston. a Lad of about 11 years of age a Son of Comfort Chappels Died with the Destemper that prevails. . .
July 18 Ester Fosdyck the Daughter of Dea Thos Fosdyck about 15 years of Age Died with the Sore Throat Distemper sick but 2 or 3 Days. all his Children Sick with it. mond 19 fair I was at home al day Lame Still Ester Fosdyck buried att Evening . . .
Aug 2 . . . Eliabeth Alley the Dauhter of Jacob Alley a young woman near 20 Died last night with the Sore Throat Distemper buried this Evening. Tuesday 3d a Rainy Day I was at home al day a girl of Jno Griffings named Eliza about 7 years old Died with the Throat Distemper . . . Thursd 19 fair & hot I was at home all day I mended 1 wheel put in 3 Spokes I borowd 1 of mr Chapman & 1 before about 2 of the Clock neighbr Thomas Truman Called up Susanna was a Dying I went over & Stayed an hour & beter She Dyed a Little past 3 of the Throat Destemper She was taken Last fryday night had been very bad at turns but yesterday was Considerably beter in a hopefull way to do well and taken in the night with a Sort of a Convulsion after She was grown worse again She was a fatt Lusty Coulered young woman about 20 yr old as likely to live as any person but a few days ago. I was at the burial this Evening Cary Latham a Child of Cary Latham Junrs above 2 year ½ old Died Son of his Second Wife Sarah Waterhouse tht was. fryd 20 fair & hot. I was at home foren. aftern. I went into Town to write a Lease for mr Treat & Chapm brot home my black mare. Saturd 21 fair most of the day a Thunder Shower toward night. I was at home al day. a Second Daughter of Jacob Alleys Dyed above 14 years of age. Sund 22 fair. Mr adams pr al dy. Ann Alleys buried toward night . . .
Sept. Saturd. 4 fair . . . Nattee was taken with the Sore throat Last night & Remains Ill all day. Sund fair Except a Small Shower . . . stayd with Nattee in the afternoon. I Sent for cuz Eliz fox who came & did wht She thot proper for him. John Savels only Son Buried near night aged 2 or 3 & a Daughter of John Colefoxes 5 years both Died with the Sore Throat Distemper yesterday. Mond 6 fair in the forenoon I was at home Looking after Nattee . . . Wednsd 15 fair . . . Ms Sarah Davise buried her youngest Daughter Margaret about 4 or 5 year old, died with the Throat Distemper. . . Tuesd 28 the Supr Court Sat. I was at Court al day My Action with Capt Wm Walker was Tryed & I finally got it. I pd the Jury 30s. & Treated ym 17s &c In the Evening Richard Christophers aged about 24 years Died taken Sick but Last fryday the 5 day. I called at his house about 9 Clock & Saw him Laid out the first man grown in Town yt died with ye Destemper. Wednsd 29 fair. I was at Court al day. Thursd 30 Rainy. I was at Court al Day. Richard Christophers buried vizt put into the Tomb. Mr Seabury pr a funeral sermon at the Church & Read over the prayers (ordained by the Church on Such occasions) at the Tomb before he was

put in. the Pall bearers were all churchmen. Hannah my Son Johns Wife was dd of a Daughter about break of day oct. 1 this night
Oct. fryd 8 fair. I was about Town foren. aftern at home Stacking ye Cornstalks & gathering 1 Ld of Pumpkins. Jno Hallam hair lip Son of Lt. Edwd Hallam aged 21 years died ys Mor. 6. Clock   Saturd 9th fair. I was about home & went to the Marshes, in the Eve at the funeral of Jno Hallam . . . Sat 16 I was at home al day fencing Stacks & mending Colln Browns Coach wheel & at the funeral of Lt Edwd Hallam who Died Last night about 3 or 4 Clock taken Last Sunday with the Throat Distemper. . . 28 fair & Cold. I was out on the Commons for Deacon Fosdick. a Child of Wm Cheapells about 11 year old buried. died with the Throat Distemper. fryd 29 fair in the foren & then Rain till night and at night Snow half Leg Deep. . .

Thus, with the exception of Groton and Stonington, where the "throat distemper" did not appear until after 1750, most of the Connecticut shore towns were involved in 1736. In an effort to check the further spread of the disease, November 24th was appointed as a "Day of Fasting and Prayer throughout the Colony,"[157] although a few of the inland towns had already become involved.

In Ridgefield, north of Stamford, there was an increase in children's deaths, although the figures are too small to be of much significance. In the east-central part of Connecticut there were frequent instances of multiple deaths.[158]   Complete figures and case descriptions are lack-

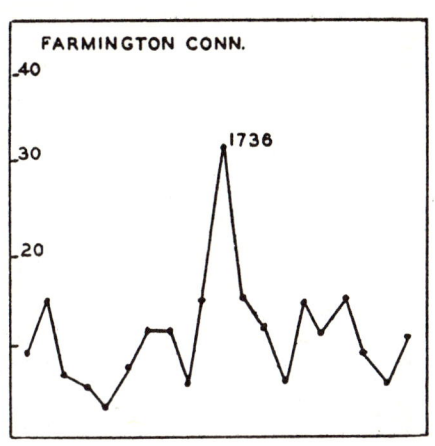

Farmington, Conn., deaths, 1726-1745.

---

[157] *Boston News-Letter*, Nov. 17-24, 1736; *Boston Evening Post*, Nov. 22, 1736.

[158] In Colchester, Ebenezer Skinner lost five children during the week ending Dec. 3, 1736. The deaths in the First Society Church Records steadily increase to reach a peak in 1740, and during 1736-40 sixty-one children died, which was about two or three times the usual number. There were multiple deaths in the Chamberlin, Dodge, Kellogg, Otis, and Pratt families. The Hebron records are too small for statistical analysis, although there were multiple deaths in the Buell, Carter, Chapwell, Ford, Newcom, and Sawyer families during 1736-40. In Lebanon, Nathan Fitch lost two in 1736; Amos Fuller lost three and Josiah Webster lost four in 1739. In East Haddam, three Brainard children died in Dec.-Jan. 1737/38, and three Gates children died in August, 1740. In Preston, there were multiple deaths in the Fobes and Witter families.

ing for these towns, but the multiple deaths alone are fair evidence of the "throat distemper" because they are seldom found anywhere in Connecticut during the ten years prior to 1736.

The epidemic appeared in Farmington somewhat earlier than in most of the inland towns and the distribution of the deaths was unusual. Asahel Strong Jr. lost four children in September, 1736, but this is the only instance of multiple deaths in the available records.[159] This relative absence of multiple deaths makes the diagnosis of "throat distemper" somewhat doubtful except for other facts. Surely there was an epidemic, as illustrated by the graph, and about eighty per cent of the excess deaths were among the children. Moreover, within a few months an epidemic began in Simsbury, the next town on the north. Here, three of the Pettibone children died in January and four of the Hays children died in March-April, 1737.[160] For a number of years Farmington and Simsbury had been relatively healthy and since some virulent childhood disease broke out in both places at about the same time, it seems fair to assume, though it is not necessarily true, that both epidemics were caused by the same disease. No case descriptions can be cited, so the disease cannot be absolutely identified but the Simsbury epidemic had all the statistical characteristics of the "throat distemper." Besides multiple deaths, there was a sudden marked increase in the death-rate and ninety-six per cent of the excess deaths during 1736-37 were among the children. If the Farmington records are complete, we may conclude that the distemper could occur without causing many multiple deaths, although it seldom appeared without them.

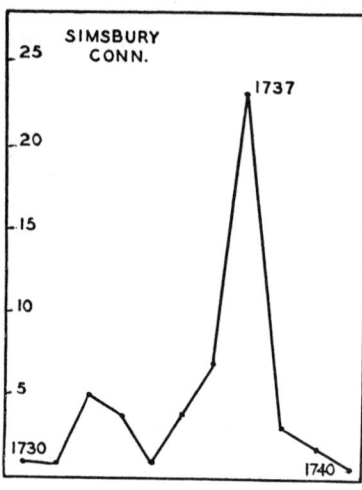

Simsbury, Conn., deaths, 1730-1740.

---

[159] The Bird, Cogswell, Cole, Denton, Gridley, Hart, Hooker, Lewis, Newel, Porter, Pratt, Seymour, Thomsen, and Woodruf families each lost a child.

[160] Albert C. Bates: *Simsbury Births, Marriages, and Deaths.* Hartford, 1898. Multiple deaths are found also in the Lampson, Holcomb, and Forward families at a later time.

The Rev. Mr. Colton of West Hartford mentioned the epidemic in his election sermon[161] before the General Assembly of 1737:

> But the common Engines of divine Wrath in the successive Ages of the World, have been Famine, Sword, and Pestilence: By these the Vengeance of an holy God has been Executed on a wicked world ...
>
> *Hence there is great reason to conclude that the people in this Land, are very much gone off from God.* For he has turned & done us hurt; He has brought many Evils upon us;
>
> *His walking contrary to us* is a sure Evidence *that we have walked contrary to Him.* If we look no farther back than the space of a Year, may we not in that Time reckon up several plain indications of the Divine displeasure? As, The *scorching Drought* of the last Summer; the *Length & extremity* of the following Winter; the *Coldness & backwardness* of the Spring and *repeated Floods,* by which much damage was sustained; but especially *that awful Sickness* that was sent among us. Of which these things are observable.
>
> 1) *Its falling mostly on Children & Young persons, by which means many, even great multitudes have been numbered to the dead.* God has inflicted on us what he threatened *Ahab* with as a heavy Judgment, 1 *King* 21 21 He has taken away our Posterity, the hope of the succeeding generation, *Rev* 2 22 There has been reason to receive that bitter lamentation *Jer* 9 21
>
> 2) The Universality of it. Not being confin'd to a few Families, not to a few Towns, or a Province; but spreading very far, even hundreds of miles.
>
> 3) *The Nature* of the *Distemper, operating with such violence, and attended with so great malignity, as to putrify the bodies (at least of some) ere the souls remove, to a degree that would (it may be) take some Weeks or Months lying in the Grave to Effect* ...

By the end of 1737, the epidemic had spread over the southern half of the colony, Newtown, Derby, and Wallingford having become involved.[162] According to the Rev. Daniel Wadworth's

---

[161] Benjamin Colton: *The Danger of Apostasie in a Sermon Preached before the General Assembly of Connecticut at Hartford, May 12th, 1737.* N. London, 1738.

[162] The Rev. Thomas Toucey of Newtown noted in his account-book the charges for treating Joseph Prindle's five children when they had the "throat distemper" (communication from Mr. Raymond J. Platt, owner of the Toucey ms.). In Derby, four children of Ephraim Washband died in Oct.-Nov. 1737, and four children of Edward Washband died in Feb. 1737/38. There were multiple deaths in the Harger and Smith families also. The Wallingford records are difficult to interpret because of marked yearly variations, but there was an increased number of children's deaths in 1737.

diary, it reached Hartford the following year:

Oct 21, 1738 . . . This day was buried a child of Sam¹ Halladays who died of yᵉ throat distemper as was supposed, and this day died a child of Daniel Seymours of yᵉ throat distemper.

He also mentions the deaths of three of Benjamin Richard's children in January, 1739, and repeatedly refers to the "time of great distress" in the fall of 1741, although he throws no light upon the nature of the disease.

On the whole, the epidemic seemed less severe throughout the colony during 1738, but the next year it started afresh, especially in the northeast towns.[163] In Coventry there was a frightful epidemic and fifty-three of the sixty-three deaths during 1739-41 were among the children, although there had been only about two deaths among the children each year for the previous twelve years.[164] Dr. Josiah Rose lost his only child. Multiple deaths were frequent and following the names of Benjamin Grover's children, the records[165] say—"all three of yᵗ Awfull Destemper in yᵉ Throt." The *New-York Weekly Journal* (Oct. 13, 1740) con-

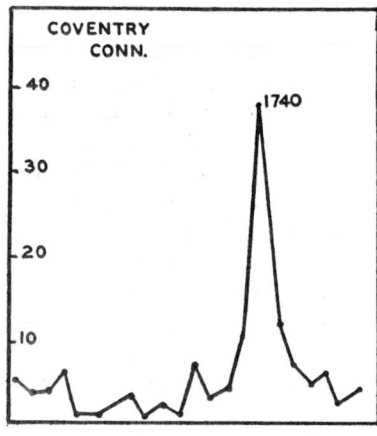

Coventry, Conn., deaths, 1725-1746.

---

[163] In Mansfield, there were multiple deaths in the Baldwin, Hall, and Sargeant families; and in Ashford, three Knowlton children died during October. John Bishop, of Bolton, lost three children in one month.

[164] S. W. Dimock: *Births, Baptisms, Marriages and Deaths in Coventry,* 1897, lists:

Name of Family	Number of Children	Dates of Death	
Rust (Daniel)	2	Aug. 15-23	1739
Grover (Benjamin)	3	Dec. 20-31	"
Skinner	2	May 7-16	1740
Carpenter	4	June 5-9	"
French	4	Aug. 2-12	"
Jones	3	Aug. 7-Sept. 8	"
Hendee	4	Aug. 27-31	"
Rust (Samuel)	3	Sept. 23-30	"
Grover (Mathew)	2	Oct. ?-Nov. ?	"
Cowls	4	July 23-Sept. 10	1741

[165] Ms. records in Conn. Hist. Soc.

tained a brief account of this epidemic:

We hear from Coventry, in Connecticut, that for several Months past the Throat Distemper has raged there in a very terrible and awful Manner; and still continues to prove exceeding mortal, even to such a Degree that by the Narrative we have had, the Plague never proved more mortal in London, and altho' application has been made to the wisest and most skilful Physicians, all Endeavors to effect a Cure prove unsuccessful and ineffectual.

Evidently the case fatality rate was very high, so diphtheria is the most probable diagnosis.

The epidemic continued to spread to the northeast and soon involved Killingly.[166] The Pomfret and Woodstock figures[167] are too small to warrant definite conclusions and, in the absence of clinical descriptions, are significant only because of an epidemic in the neighboring towns.

The total number of deaths in Connecticut can only be roughly estimated, since no figures are available for Fairfield, Glastonbury, Stratford, Wethersfield, and Windsor, and the records for Hartford, New Haven, New London, and Stamford are obviously incomplete. The records of

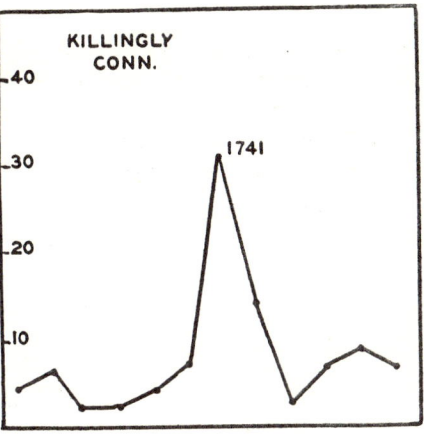

Killingly, Conn., deaths, 1735-1746.

[166] Name of Family	Number of Children	Dates of Deaths	
Cabot	3	Nov. 11-22	1740
Child	2	Oct. 24-Nov. 5	"
Dresser	3	Jan. 1-14	1741
Morse	3	April 17-May 11	"
Whitmore (Daniel)	5	May 1-June 5	"
Whitmore	4	June 1-20	"
Bixby	2	Sept. 26-Oct. 4	"
Sterns	3	Sept. 16-Oct. 20	"
Upham	4	Sept. 27-Oct. 15	"

[167] There were slight increases in children's deaths in 1736 and 1739. Two Martin children died in 1736 and two Morries children died in 1739; there were no other multiple deaths.

a few towns are of interest:

Town	Estimated population[168]	Epidemic years	Excess number of deaths	Per cent under 20 years
Coventry	800	1739–41	54	87
East Haven	200	1736–37	26	100
Farmington	1800	1736	24	80
Guilford	1100	1736	44	82
Killingly	1000	1740–42	46	90
Simsbury	1100	1736–37	29	96
	6000		223	Aver. 92

The variation in the percentages under twenty years can be partly attributed to the method of estimation. The ratio of deaths to population (37 per 1000) cannot be used to estimate the total number of deaths in the colony, because there is little evidence of an epidemic in the northwest and southeast parts and because some towns within the path of the epidemic (Branford and

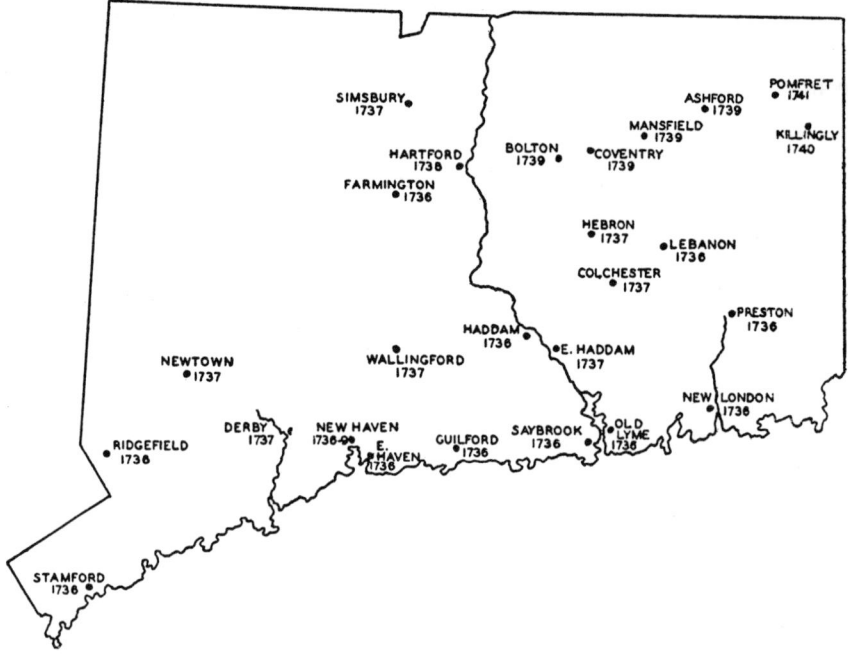

The spread of the epidemic throughout the towns of Connecticut.

---

[168] Approximately one-half of the census figures for 1756, by which time the colony had doubled in population.

Killingworth, for example) had no increase in deaths although the records seem to be complete. By actual count over five hundred deaths can be attributed to the epidemic and if the records were complete the number would probably approach one thousand.

It is impossible to estimate the relative importance of scarlet fever and diphtheria in Connecticut, because there is very little clinical information at hand. The "Rash" that was present in East Guilford in 1740 was probably scarlet fever, therefore that disease was probably present in many other towns. Also, in some towns such as Colchester, Hebron, East Haddam, and Woodstock, the deaths were irregularly distributed with increases occurring in separate years and this irregular distribution may have been caused by the presence of two diseases. As has been said, Marblehead (Mass.) had two epidemics very close together but caused by different diseases; the Harvard and Cambridge records suggest a mild epidemic in 1736, possibly scarlet fever, and a second more serious epidemic in 1739-40, possibly diphtheria. It is only because a few Connecticut towns show somewhat analogous findings that two diseases are suspected. The sustained or double peak, however, may be explained on the basis of a single disease. Within the geographical limits of many towns there were two or more separate church societies which were often very far apart and the disease could appear in one and then not in the other until a much later date. To some extent, the spread of the disease would depend upon the treatment by the town physician, for if he believed that the disease was contagious, he might have temporarily inhibited the spread, although on account of the unsuspected healthy carriers he could not have stopped it altogether. So, if separate parts of a town became involved at different times, the records would reveal an irregular rise because all the names were recorded in the same book and it is impossible to determine where each family lived.

Even if scarlet fever was prevalent in Connecticut, there is no reason to suppose that it was any more serious than elsewhere at the same time. The records of Boston, Marblehead, Guilford (?), New York, and New Jersey, the only places where one can be certain that scarlet fever was present to any great extent, indicate that at that time it was a comparatively mild disease and did not greatly contribute to the total mortality of the "throat distemper."

Although it is possible that scarlet fever alone or in combination with diphtheria may have caused some of the trouble in a few Connecticut towns, the evidence suggests that, on the whole, the epidemic was caused by a single disease, which first appeared in the southwest (Stamford, 1736) and spread gradually to the northeast (Killingly, 1740-41). The Stamford clinical evidence, the frequency of multiple deaths in nearly all of the towns, and the very high mortality in Coventry and some of the other towns make a diagnosis of diphtheria more than probable.

True recurrences of the epidemic occurred in many Connecticut towns, as elsewhere in New England (see Hampton graph). These recurrences appeared some five to ten years later but they were too irregular and too numerous for a detailed account.

IX

NEW YORK

No effort has been made to trace the epidemic in New York. Cadwallader Colden supposed that it spread directly from Kingston and that it took two years to reach the Hudson River:[169]

It continued on the east side of Hudson's river, before it passed to the west, and appeared in those places, to which the people of New England chiefly resorted for trade, and in the places through which they travelled.

He also intimated that the disease was mild when accompanied by a rash and was more fatal when the larynx was involved. Here again there is evidence of both diseases, but most of Colden's information was obtained through correspondence with William Douglass and it is impossible to determine the part that can be attributed to personal observation.

The epidemic appeared on Long Island also. The Rev. Ebenezer Prime noted in his diary:[170]

On October 3d, 1736, after a short but violent Illness, dyed at Huntington, of the throat distemper, my dear sister Hannah Prime.

The disease probably spread to Huntington from Stamford, which is directly across the sound. In Easthampton, also, there were many deaths from the distemper during 1736 and 1738.[171]

---

[169] *Med. Obs. and Inquiries*, 1753, i, 211.
[170] E. D. G. Prime: *Notes of the Prime Family*. 1888, p. 20.
[171] *N. Y. Geneal. & Biog. Rec.*, xxxiv, 251.

X

NEW JERSEY

> To th' silent Grave, great numbers have,
> of late been carried,
> Our Children dear, both far and near,
> are posting to the dead.
> —Earnest Expostulation.

An account of the New England epidemic would be incomplete without reference to a similar one in New Jersey because it is possible that they were related to each other.

On February 9, 1735/6, the *New York Weekly Journal* reported an epidemic of "Throat Distemper" at Crosswicks in West Jersey. A clinical description of the "terrible Disease in the Throat that has made such Desolations in the Country" appeared the following week in the same journal. The anonymous author said that the epidemic began "at Newark Mountains [Orange]; and at first proved mortal to almost all that had it." In his description there are indications of diphtheria of the throat and larynx, but although there are also indications of tonsillitis and some extraneous diseases, no evidence of scarlet fever can be discerned. This article, though unsigned, was written by the Rev. Jonathan Dickinson (1688-1747).[172] He, Jared Eliot, another notable minister-physician of Killingworth, and Timothy Woodbridge, a minister at Simsbury, comprised the class of 1706 at Yale. Two years later, he was called to the church at Elizabeth Town, New Jersey; and eventually he became the first president of the College of New Jersey (Princeton). Those were the days when theological questions were settled by pamphlet wars, and Dickinson, with a courageous and prolific pen, became generally known as one of the ablest and most influential religious leaders in the colonies.[173]

Dickinson's second medical work, more notable than his first, was entitled: *Observations on that terrible Disease vulgarly called the Throat Distemper* . . . It was dated at Elizabeth Town, Feb. 20, 1738/9 and printed in Boston in 1740. This pamphlet,

---

[172] "In my No 119, I inserted a Letter from Mr. Jonathan Dickinson of Elizabeth-Town, containing an Account and proposing a Method of Cure of a Distemper which rages in divers Parts of this Country." *New-York Weekly Journal*, March 8, 1735/36.

[173] E. F. Hatfield: *Hist. of Elizabeth.* 1868, p. 326.

CXIX.

THE
New-York Weekly JOURNAL.

Containing the freshest Advices, Foreign, and Domestick.

MUNDAY February 16th, 1735.

Mr. Zenger.

THE following Letter contains a particular Discription of a fatal Distemper, which is now epidemical in many Parts of this Country; proposes a Method of Cure, which has been attended with uncommon Success, if you'll give it a Place in your Journal, it may gratify many of your Readers, and be of extensive Service to Mankind.

A Letter to a Friend in New-York.

SIR,

According to your Desire, I shall endeavour to give you the most plain and familiar Account I can of the terrible Disease in the Throat, that has made such Desolations in the Country; with the Method of Cure that has proved so very successful in these Parts, that there has few or none dyed under my Care for a great while, that I could seasonably and steadily tend; except some that would not be perswaded, and were so Old to be compelled to the necessary Methods of cleansing their Throats.

The Disease began near a Year ago at *Newark* Mountains; and at first proved Mortal to almost all that had it; and has continued among us ever since, that I have had great Opportunity of a particular Acquaintance with it; and great Cause of Thankfulness for a continued Series of Success, in dealing with it.

It's common Appearance is with a Tumefaction of the *Tonsils, Uvula,* and Parts adjacent, which at first appear very red and enflamed; and, in about two or three Days, and sometimes sooner, are covered with a white Furr, very easily washed off at first; but if not immediately cleansed and kept clean, it fastens, grows hard, and can no way be removed, but by a gradual Digestion, whereby it is loosened, and comes off like an Escar. It ordinarily extends to the *Larynx* or Mouth of the *Windpipe*, and so finishes the Tragedy, by taking away the Voice, and procuring a continual ringing Cough.

It sometimes raises the Cuticula upon the *Tonsils, Uvula,* and contiguous Parts; and appears with Pustules, greatly resembling the separate *Small-Pox,* filled with a laudable Coloured Pus, and this we find the most favourable Kind.

It sometimes appears with a small Pimple, Blister or Scab, upon the Face or Neck, from whence a speedy and large Inflammation arises in all the adjacent Parts, very much imitating an *Erisipelas,* which soon seizes the inside of the Throat, and if not immediately helped, terminates in a mortal Gangreen.

It very often begins behind the *Ears,* in the *Armpits,* upon the *Navil* or other Parts of the Body, at first with a white Protuberance, the neighbouring Parts enflaming and encreasing to a great Bigness with a swelling and quickly turning Black and sphacelating, if not prevented. If these corrosive Ulcers are seasonably cured, it usually prevents the sore Throat, it otherwise commonly finishes there.

It often appears in the Form of a *Bubo,* or very angry *Boil,* under the Ears, behind the Head or upon the Neck, which if quick digested and opened, the Patient is safe, otherwise a Mortal Gangreen may ensue.

If the Disease gains Ground, and is not seasonably checked, the Glands quite round the Neck are much swelled, and the whole Neck is covered with Tumors about the bigness of a Nutmegg; and the Tumefaction sometimes extends even to the Pit of the Stomack.

Th

(Courtesy of the New York Public Library.)

the second medical publication by a Yale graduate,[174] is one of the few outstanding contributions to early American medicine and since it is now very scarce, yet of great importance in the history of the "throat distemper," a few of the essential passages are quoted at length:[175]

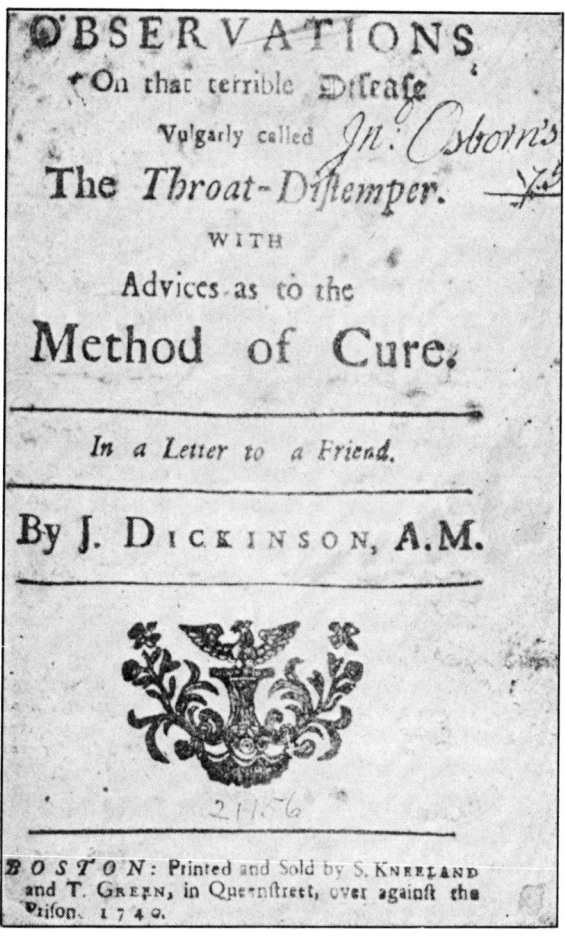

(Courtesy of the New York Academy of Medicine.)

This Distemper first began in these Parts, in Febr. 1734/5. The long Continuance and universal Spread of it among us, has given me abundant Opportunity to be acquainted with it in all its Forms.

The first Assault was in a Family about ten Miles from me, which proved fatal to eight of the Children in about a Fortnight. Being called to visit the distressed Family, I found upon my arrival, one of the Children newly dead, which gave me the Advantage of a Dissection, and thereby a better Acquaintance with the Nature of the Disease, than I could otherwise have had: . . .

The above is quoted, not only because of the importance of the date and multiple deaths, but also to show that Dickinson had the qualifications of a true physician. It is doubtful if any other con-

---

[174] The first was John Walton's *Essay on Fevers, the Rattles and Canker.* Boston, 1732.

[175] From a reprint in Wickes: *Hist. of Med. in New Jersey.* 1879, p. 87 et seq.

temporary minister displayed such a desire for medical knowledge as to bother with an autopsy. In an orderly manner, he then proceeds to a description of the disease and mentions a "variety of types":

1. I take this Disease to be naturally an Eruptive milliary Fever: and when it appears as such, it usually begins with a Shivering, a Chill, or with Stretching, or Yawning; which is quickly succeeded with a sore Throat, a Tumefaction of the Tonsils, Uvula and Epiglottis, and sometimes of the Jaws, and even of the whole Throat and Neck. The Fever is often acute, the Pulse quick and high and the Countenance florid. The Tonsils first, and in a little Time the whole Throat covered with a whitish Crustula, the Tongue furr'd, and the Breath fetid. Upon the 2d, 3d, or 4th Day, if proper Methods are used, the Patient is cover'd with a milliary Eruption, in some exactly resembling the Measels, in others more like the Scarlet Fever (for which Distemper it has frequently been mistaken) but in others it very much resembles the confluent Small Pox. When the Eruption is finished, the Tumefaction every where subsides, the Fever abates, and the Slough in the Throat casts off and falls. The Eruption often disappears about the 6th or 7th Day; tho' it sometimes continues visible much longer. After the Eruption is over, the Cuticle scales and falls off, as in the Conclusion of the Scarlet Fever. If after the Cure of this Disease Purging be neglected, the Sick may seem to recover Health & Strength for a while; yet they frequently in a little Time fall again into grievous Disorders; such as a great prostration of Strength, loss of Appetite, hectical Appearances, sometimes great Dissiness of Sight, and often such a weakness in the Joints as deprives them of the Use of all their Limbs; and some of them are affected with scorbutick Symptoms of almost every Kind.

When this Distemper appears in the Form now described, it is not very dangerous: I have seldom seem any die with it, unless by a sudden Looseness, that calls in the Eruptions, or by some very irregular Treatment.

Even though there is some suggestion of diphtheria, and even in spite of his specific denial, Dickinson was undoubtedly dealing with the disease that we now call scarlet fever. It is also apparent that the New Jersey scarlet fever was, as a rule, comparatively mild.

But there are several other very different Appearances of the Disease, which are attended with more frightful and deadly Consequences.

2. It frequently begins with a slight Indisposition, much resembling an ordinary Cold, with a listless Habit, a slow & scarce discernable Fever, some soreness of the Throat and Tumefaction of the Tonsils: and perhaps a running of the Nose, the Countenance pale, and the eyes dull and heavy. The Patient is not confin'd, nor any Danger apprehended for some Days, till the

Fever gradually increases, the whole Throat, and sometimes the Roof of the Mouth and Nostrils, are covered with a cankerous Crust, which corrodes the contiguous Parts, and frequently terminates in a mortal Gangreen, if not by seasonable Applications prevented. The Stomach is sometimes, and the Lungs often, covered with the same Crustula... When the Lungs are thus affected, the Patient is first afflicted with a dry hollow Cough, which is quickly succeeded with an extraordinary Hoarseness and total Loss of the Voice, with the most distressing asthmatic Symptoms and difficulty of Breathing, under which the poor miserable Creature struggles, until released by a perfect Suffocation, or Stoppage of the Breath. This last has been the fatal Symptom, under which the most have sunk, that have died in these parts. And indeed there have comparatively but few recovered, whose Lungs have been thus affected. All that I have seen to get over this dreadful Symptom... have by their perpetual Cough expectorated incredible Quantities of a tough whitish Slough from their Lungs, for a considerable Time together. And on the other Hand, I have seen large Pieces of this Crust, several Inches long and near an Inch broad, torn from the Lungs by the vehemence of the Cough, without any Signs of Digestion, or possibility of obtaining it.

This could not have been any disease other than diphtheria and obviously Dickinson must have seen many cases to write such an excellent description. His types three and five, however, are neither scarlet fever nor diphtheria, whereas type four is diphtheria of the skin. His sixth and last type is uncomplicated laryngeal diphtheria:

6. This Disease appears sometimes in the Form of a Quinsey. The Lungs are inflamed, the Throat and especially the Epiglottis exceedingly tumefied. In a few Hours the Sick is brought to the Height of an Orthopnœa; and cannot breathe but in an erect Posture, and then with great Difficulty and Noise. This may be distinguished from an Angina, by the Crustula in the Throat, which determines it to be a Sprout from the same Root with the Symptoms described above. In this Case the Patient sometimes dies in twenty-four hours. I have not seen any one survive the third Day. But thro' the Divine Goodness these Symptoms have been more rarely seen among us, and there have been but few in this Manner snatch'd out of the World.

Dickinson, trained for the ministry, had more clinical ability than most of the physicians of his time. He had the two diseases clearly separated in his mind, and was also aware of the difference in mortality. Concerning the second group of cases (diphtheria), he said that "all attempts to bring out the milliary eruptions seem in vain." In Boston, this would have been considered a confession of therapeutic ignorance. Unlike most of his contemporaries, he was ready to admit his limitations: "I have not yet found any effectual Remedy in the 6th and last Case described." Apparently his medical knowledge was acquired through independent and intelligent observation and if he had not attempted to square his facts with the accepted theories of the day, he would very probably have ended the confusion of scarlet fever with diphtheria and thus would have made a great contribution to the medical literature of the world. But unfortunately he, like William Douglass, insisted that the various types were different manifestations of one disease, which was naturally accompanied by a rash, and his first intention was "to bring out the Eruption as soon as possible." He saw patients who had both diseases at different times and he thought they were second attacks of the same disease, although he added: "I have never seen any upon whom the Eruptions could be brought out more than once."

In 1738, Dickinson went to Boston and talked with "several gentlemen" who were particularly interested in this epidemic. It cannot definitely be said that he met William Douglass, but it is more than probable that these two distinguished physicians actually met and exchanged ideas, since each reflects the influence of the other in their later works. In his first contribution to *Zenger's Weekly* in February, 1736, Dickinson did not include scarlet fever in his description, but in his *Observations* (1740), which were written after he had been to Boston, he embodies Douglass' opinion that scarlet fever and diphtheria were the same disease; he also frequently uses Douglass' term "Eruptive Milliary Fever." On the other hand, Douglass, in his *Practical History* (1736) describes chiefly scarlet fever and denies the possibility of a second attack, but in his letter to Colden (1739) he admits the frequency of "Second Seizures" and stresses the occurrence of diphtheritic croup,—ideas that may have been suggested by Dickinson. Both firmly believed in the "morbific matter" theory and in the importance of bringing out the rash.

Eighteenth century physicians had a good excuse for believing in the identity of the two diseases because, after all, the diseases are somewhat similar. Moreover, diphtheria is a disease that may become evident in many different ways. One patient may appear to have a simple "cold in the head"; another, some affection of the skin; and a third may suffocate within a few hours. Now, if a single disease can manifest itself in so many different ways, is it faulty judgment to suppose that it might also cause a scarlet rash? The chief criticism, if any, is that both Dickinson and Douglass displayed the very human fault of confusing hearsay with fact. I do not think that Douglass would have confused the two diseases if he had actually observed the early New Hampshire cases. He was told about the New Hampshire disease and, without personal investigation, believed it was the same as the one in Boston. Similarly, I do not think that Dickinson would have included his "variety of types" in an all-inclusive whole if he had not been influenced by Douglass, or by someone else in Boston, who probably told him that the diseases were the same. Both men merely reflected the prevailing theories of their time. The identity of diseases originated long before the eighteenth century, and was in vogue even as late as 1796 when Charles Caldwell, a student at the University of Pennsylvania, inadvertently reduced the theory to absurdity in his graduating thesis upon "the original sameness" of water on the brain, membranous croup, and infantile diarrhea!

In relation to the New England epidemic, the important facts as told by Dickinson are: that an epidemic appeared in New Jersey in February, 1735, which was three months before the New Hampshire outbreak; that it was chiefly an epidemic of diphtheria; that this epidemic also was complicated by the presence of scarlet fever; and that the scarlet fever, like the scarlet fever in New England, was comparatively mild.

XI

COMMENT

> And yet we must such Notice take,
> That we may right Improvement make, . . .
> —An Elegy.

The reactions of different populations to various diseases often reveal important facts which help in the control of future epidemics, and for that reason a study of the "throat distemper" records may be worth while. In many respects this epidemic was unique. There had been epidemics of whooping cough, measles, smallpox, dysentery, and influenza in the colonies, but they were more limited in extent and time, whereas this epidemic extended over nearly all the inhabited regions of New England, lasted many years, and was supposed to have been a new disease on virgin soil. Moreover, uncontrolled diphtheria epidemics do not occur today, and, one sincerely hopes, will never be observed again. Unfortunately for a scientific analysis, however, the "throat distemper" was a complicated epidemic. It has already been shown that it consisted of a scarlet fever and two separate diphtheria epidemics and, furthermore, that what the colonists thought was a new disease was probably nothing new at all. Therefore, although these records may not reveal any facts of very great importance, nevertheless, I believe they have some scientific value.

— 1 —

Whether or not diphtheria and scarlet fever existed in New England prior to 1735 has much importance in the interpretation of the records, so it is well to assemble all available evidence in an effort to arrive at some conclusion. The fragmentary history of those diseases does not allow one to say with certainty when each was first observed, and the available descriptions are often so brief that it is hazardous even to attempt a differential diagnosis. If either disease was mild it may have been present from earliest times and, like the common cold, mumps, and chicken pox, may not have seemed unusual enough to elicit comment. Also, the old records are often difficult to evaluate. Sometimes the accounts were noticeably exaggerated, as when the *New York Gazette* reported that the Coventry "throat distemper" was more mortal than the London plague; on the contrary, frightful epidemics sometimes received scant notice. There would be nothing known about the Haverhill epidemic, for instance, except for the Rev. John Brown,—the town records of that period are more concerned with such things as the rum distillery and the ferry and the boundary perambulations. In many other towns, the only evidence of an epidemic is concealed in the vital records which, of course, were never kept for statistical purposes. So it is mostly by chance that we know anything about colonial diseases and the proof that a disease existed often rests upon the most casual and indirect statements.

There is some evidence of a diphtheria epidemic throughout New England as early as 1659. According to Cotton Mather:[176]

---

[176] *Magnalia* (1702 edit.) Bk. IV, iii, 156. Danforth himself gives a slightly different version: "1659. 9^m & 10^m. The Lord sent a general visitation of children by coughs & colds, of wch my 3 children Sarah, Mary & Elisabeth Danforth died, all of y^m within ye space of a fortnight." *N. Engl. Hist. & Geneal. Reg.*, 1880, xxxiv, 87. Whooping cough was also present in 1659 (Hull's Diary), but I do not believe that the two diseases were confused. Whooping cough was not as fatal as the "Bladders" and besides was not "unknown."

THE "THROAT DISTEMPER" OF 1735-1740

In *December* 1659, the (until then unknown) Malady of *Bladders in the Windpipe*, invaded and removed many Children; by Opening of one of them the Malady and Remedy (too late for many) were discovered. Among those many that thereby expired, were the Three Children of the Reverend Mr. Samuel Danforth . . .

Bladders or rattles in the throat or windpipe were the old terms for what is now called "croup" and so the Danforth children very probably had diphtheria which is generally the cause of the most serious form of croup. The Rowley records show some evidence of an epidemic during 1659-60 characterized by multiple deaths of children.[177] At about the same time, "Cynanche Trachealis," which was an old technical term for croup, was present in Connecticut and in 1662 the General Assembly declared a day of thanksgiving for deliverance from the affliction.[178] Josselyn[179] mentions in his description of New England:

Also they are troubled with a disease in the mouth or throat which hath proved mortal to some in a very short time, Quinsies, and Impostumations of the Almonds [tonsils], with great distempers of cold.

There were many deaths in New London during 1689 from a "Distemper of sore throats and ffeaver . . . the Like haveing not been knowne in ye Memory of man" but the exact nature of the disease is uncertain.[180] In 1693, Sir Francis Wheeler arrived at Boston with his fleet. He had left England on an expedition to drive the French from North America, but when he reached the West Indies the crew contracted some disease and the expedition failed. The epidemic continued aboard ship and on reaching Boston, the fleet was quarantined; nevertheless the disease gained a foothold in the town. Samuel Sewall and Cotton Mather both mention the event and subsequent historians have assumed that this disease was yellow fever, but the Rev. John Barnard says in his autobiography that he was a boy at that time and contracted the disease and that it was scarlet fever.[181] Not too much emphasis should be placed upon Barnard's boyhood recollections yet his use

---

[177] *First Book of Burialls of the Town of Rowley. Essex Inst. Hist. Coll.* v, p. 161.

[178] Quoted from Packard: *Hist. of Med. in U. S.* (1931).

[179] Josselyn: *Account of Two Voyages. Coll. Mass. Hist. Soc.* 1883, 3rd Ser., iii, p. 333.

[180] Caulkins: *Hist. of New London.*

[181] *Coll. Mass. Hist. Soc.*, 3rd Ser., v, p. 181.

of the words "scarlet fever" may mean that the disease was known, at least, in 1693. The first reliable evidence of scarlet fever that I can find is Cotton Mather's mention[182] of a Boston epidemic in 1702. The same epidemic may have spread to other towns, for that year in Salisbury, a son of the Rev. John Pike died "after two days Relapse into a fever his principal malady was sore throat and caput-dolor."[183] Three of Mather's children had scarlet fever in 1704. "Throat Distemper" is supposed to have been present in Amesbury during the summer of 1706 when a Mrs. Weed and her three children all died on the same day, but the evidence is not convincing.[184] There was an epidemic in Connecticut during 1712 which may partly have been diphtheria, for in Woodbury two of Joseph Judson's children died "of a bladder in the throat as is supposed."[185] A childhood disease accompanied by multiple deaths was present in Mansfield (Conn.) during 1726-27, and about the same time in New London, a child of four years "died with a distemper in the throat."[186] During 1728-29, the Rowley records show an epidemic with multiple deaths and other characteristics of the throat distemper. There was a small epidemic of some virulent childhood disease in Braintree (Mass.) during 1730-31, which may have been either scarlet fever or diphtheria.[187] In nearby Dedham one or both of those diseases probably caused the trouble in the Rev. Samuel Dexter's family:[188]

Decr 10th 1729, ab^t this Time all three of my Children were visited with ye Quincey—two of them very bad, but y^{ey} were none of 'em delivered over unto death . . . Nov. 5th 1731. My third Son, John, Dyed ab^t 6 of ye Clock in ye Evening, after a few Days very distressing Indisposition, being taken so very ill on ye Tuesday & dyed on ye fryday following of ye Canker, &c. He was a most pleasant & Desireable Child. . . Feb^{ry} 2d 1734-5, at ab^t ½ hour past four in ye Morning, Died of ye Squinancy, my Dear & only Daughter, Catherina, aged sixteen Months & five Days. She was a very pleasant & Desireable Child, & had a very Awful & Shocking Death. . .

In Norwich, diphtheria may have caused the deaths of Benjamin Lothrop's three children in December, 1732; the same disease was

---

[182] *Diary of Cotton Mather.* Coll. Mass. Hist. Soc., 7th Ser., pp. 446, 454.
[183] *Coll. New Hamp. Hist. Soc.,* iii, p. 43.
[184] Joseph Merrill: *Hist. of Amesbury.* 1880, p. 157.
[185] Barnes: *Mortality Record of Woodbury.* 1898.
[186] *Diary of Joshua Hempstead.* Published by the New London Hist. Soc.
[187] Samuel A. Bates: *Records of the Town of Braintree,* p. 729.
[188] *Samuel Dexter's Diary.* loc. cit.

present in the Stratfield Society (Bridgeport) during October, 1733, when Eunice Beardslee and Edward Burrows both died "of ye Bladder aged 1 year."[189] In the "throat distemper" records we find lay writers frequently mentioning scarlet fever, which can be taken as indirect evidence that that disease had been very common before 1735. The newspapers reported scarlet fever at Ipswich; Douglass said that some of the New Hampshire cases were "called a scarlet fever"; and John Brown mentioned scarlet fever in connection with some Haverhill deaths. At each occurrence it was not described as a new disease but merely mentioned in terms which indicate that the public must have been very familiar with it.

In summary, we can be certain that diphtheria was present in the colonies for many years and sometimes in serious epidemic form, particularly in Massachusetts and Connecticut, but not enough records are available to make definite statements about its presence in New Hampshire. Scarlet fever was present, certainly in Massachusetts and probably in New Hampshire, but I have found no early records of it in Connecticut. Its relative mildness may be the probable explanation for its being seldom mentioned. It may have become more fatal during 1735–40, but even then it was mild in comparison with diphtheria and, except as a cause of diagnostic confusion, was not a major factor in the "throat distemper" epidemic.

— 2 —

The previous existence of diphtheria may partly explain the different death-rates in the separate provinces:

Province	Estimated population[190]	Epidemic years	Total deaths	Deaths per 1000 population
New Hampshire	20,000	1735–36	1,000	
		1736–40	500	75.0
Maine	9,000	1735–40	500	55.5
Massachusetts	130,000	1735–40	2,000	15.4
Connecticut	63,000	1735–40	1,000	15.8
	222,000		5,000	22.5

The New Hampshire death-rate is based upon Fitch's figures and also upon the easily proven fact that the epidemic continued

---
[189] Ms. records in Conn. State Library.
[190] Estimates from Damon's *American Dict. of Dates*. Boston, 1921, Vol. i.

long after the "Account" was published, not only in the frontier towns but also in Portsmouth and its vicinity. The deaths can be attributed almost entirely to diphtheria. On account of geographical proximity, time relation, and the frequency of multiple deaths, the Maine epidemic was very probably a continuation of the New Hampshire one and therefore an epidemic of diphtheria also, even though specific disease descriptions are not available. The number of deaths, included here merely for completeness, is taken from Williamson, who probably did not use actual statistics but made estimates based upon comparative populations and Fitch's records of New Hampshire deaths. The Massachusetts epidemic, as has been said, was very complicated and many deaths were caused by scarlet fever. It has been estimated that there were 1400 deaths in Essex County alone and 2000 deaths in the whole province, which I believe are the minimum figures, but since it is impossible to estimate the scarlet fever deaths, the Massachusetts figures are therefore disregarded. The reasons for attributing most of the Connecticut deaths to diphtheria have been given elsewhere. The search for records of an epidemic in Rhode Island has been unsuccessful.[191] Connecticut and Massachusetts towns near the Rhode Island boundaries (Groton, Stonington, Killingly, Uxbridge) were not involved until 1740 or later, so Rhode Island was probably not involved until a later date. In 1738, the Rhode Island laws concerning contagious distempers were modified but that may have been merely a precautionary measure.

To simplify the present discussion, only New Hampshire and Connecticut are compared. In proportion to population, the New Hampshire epidemic was a great deal more severe; according to the figures there were five times as many deaths. The difference becomes apparent also by comparing the separate towns. In very few Connecticut towns was the mortality as great as that in Durham,

---

[191] Between May 10 and June 7, 1736, the widow Carey of Bristol lost six children; and there were two deaths in Capt. Lawton's family during July. See: *Vital Records of Rhode Island 1636-1850*, Vol. v, 122. Also: *Boston News-Letter*, May 27-June 3, 1736. I can find no other evidence of an epidemic. John Walton in *The Religion of Jesus Vindicated* (1736, p. 26) says: ". . . His Rod has had a loud Voice in New-England this last Year; Oh! How many have been suddenly called into the eternal World by a late raging Distemper, and especially among young People?" This does not necessarily refer to Rhode Island, although the author practised medicine there. Walton also mentions in a letter, dated 1744, that the "throat distemper" was present in Glocester, R. I.

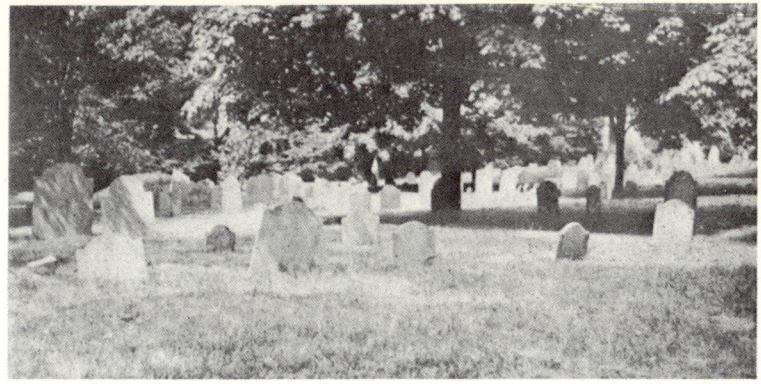

Gravestones of the children of Samuel and Mary Upham;—Phebe, Abigail, William, and Marcy,—who died between August 15 and September 14, 1738. Malden, Mass.

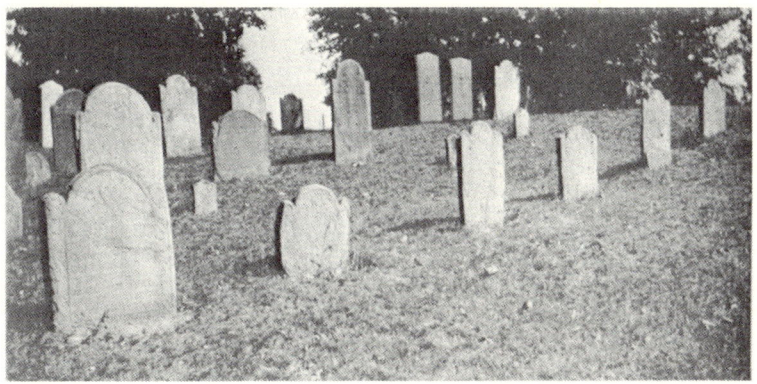

Gravestones of Mrs. Martha Gott and her five children,—Nathaniel, died October 29; Rebekah, died November 14; Martha, died November 15; John, died November 29; Josiah, died December 5, 1737. Wenham, Mass.

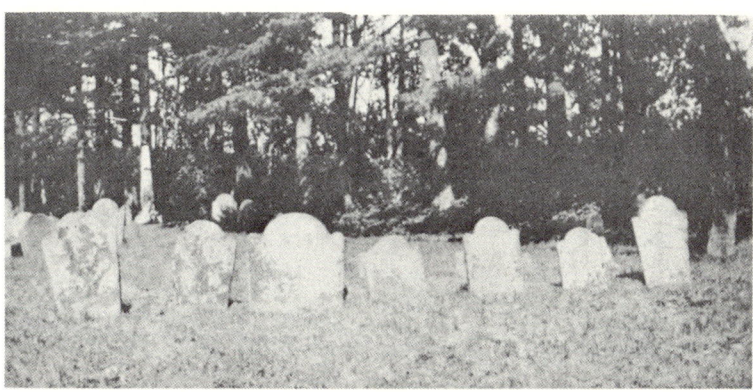

Gravestones of the children of Joseph and Rebeckah Moor;—Ephraim, aged 7, died June 15; Hannah, aged 3, died June 17; Jacob, aged 11, died June 18 (all three buried in one grave); Cathorign, aged 2, died June 23; Rebeckah, aged 6, died June 26; and Lucy, aged 14, died August 22, 1740. Lancaster, Mass. Old **Common Burial Ground.**

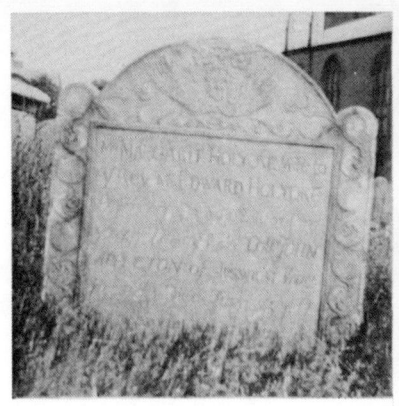 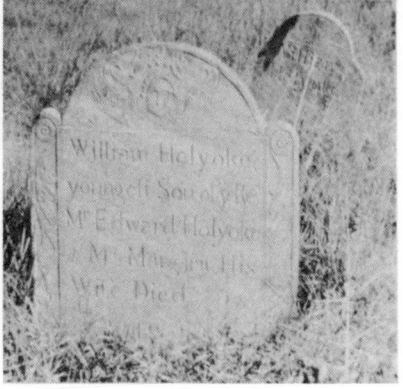

Gravestones of Mrs Margarit Holyoke and of William Holyoke. Cambridge, Mass., 1740.

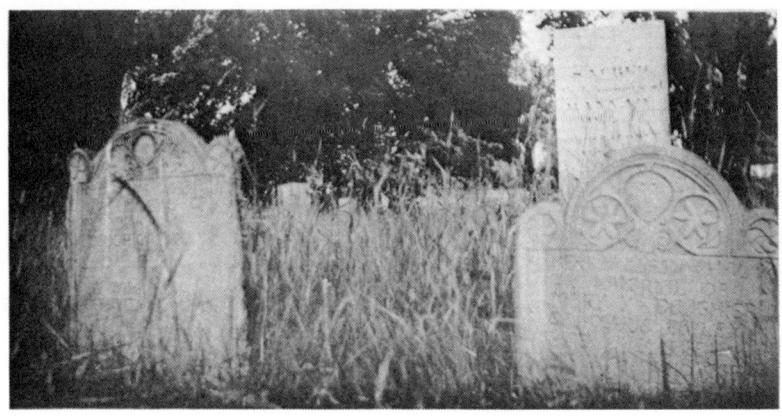

Gravestones of Elizabeth and Mary Bayley. Haverhill, Mass., May, 1736.

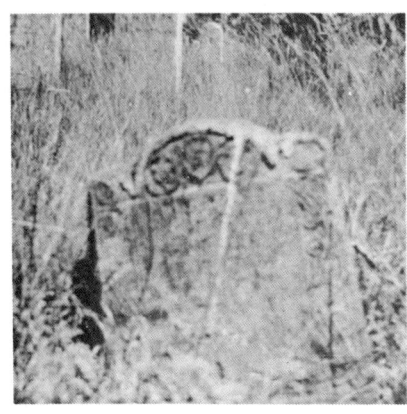

Gravestone of David Greley, who died June 20, 1735, aged 11 years. One of the first victims of the epidemic. Kingston, N. H.

Gravestones of Stephen Mix, aged 9, died May 21, 1736; and Mary Mix, aged 4, died June 11, 1736. New Haven, Conn.

Hampton Falls, Kingston, or Rye and one gathers the impression from contemporary comments and the somewhat greater frequency of multiple deaths that, regardless of any figures, the New Hampshire epidemic caused more destruction. This marked difference in mortality can be explained in at least two ways. First, contrary to contemporary opinion, it now appears that the Connecticut epidemic was not an integral part of the epidemic that began in Kingston. The Connecticut epidemic appeared in Stamford and towns along the shore and later spread to the northeast corner of the colony. In other words, it spread towards Massachusetts and New Hampshire, whereas if New England was involved in a single epidemic the course should have been in the opposite direction because epidemics usually spread away from the original source. So, unless we adopt the explanation that the disease was carried from the "Eastward" towns around Cape Cod to the towns on the Connecticut shore, it seems necessary to assume that the Connecticut epidemic either was a part of the New Jersey epidemic, or, like the one in New Jersey, had an independent origin. If the Connecticut disease was caused by a less virulent type of diphtheria, the difference in mortality can be readily explained.

It is also possible to explain this difference in mortality on the basis of a difference in immunity. The history of diphtheria in New England prior to 1735 suggests that the disease had been more common in Connecticut and this may have had a lasting effect upon the population. Recent laboratory experiments indicate that the progeny of mice that have recovered from certain diseases are more resistant to the same diseases than are the progeny of unselected mice[192] and therefore the Connecticut children may have been more immune because of inheritance. Moreover, it is supposed that the proportion of immune subjects in a given population varies with the incidence of the disease, and, if it can be assumed that diphtheria was common in Connecticut and uncommon in New Hampshire, the difference in mortality can again be readily explained. But it is not at all certain that diphtheria was uncommon in New Hampshire before this epidemic. The absence of records does not mean the absence of the disease; nevertheless, the assumption that there were immunity differences among various populations seems to be justified on other grounds. Throughout the whole history of the "throat distemper," one finds evidence that the disease was more fatal in

---

[192] L. T. Webster. *Experimental Epidemiology. Medicine*, 1932, xi, 321.

the smaller frontier towns. In proportion to their populations, Kingston and Durham suffered more than Exeter; Hampton Falls more than Hampton; Rye and the Shoals more than Portsmouth; Byfield more than Newbury; Coventry and Simsbury more than Hartford; East Haven more than New Haven; and so on with other groups of towns. With the exception of Haverhill and Kittery—two old established towns with frightful epidemics—the smaller frontier towns generally bore the brunt of the attack. Epidemiologists have observed a difference in the reactions of rural and urban populations to disease and though it should be remembered that all of these towns possessed rural populations and the only essential differences were in size and age, some similar difference in population reactions seems to have been present. If it can be assumed, for instance, that diphtheria had been constantly present in the old established towns, even in New Hampshire, and had left some immunity effect, we have a possible explanation for the various differences in mortality. Connecticut at that time possessed more old established towns and was less of a frontier colony than was New Hampshire.

Whatever the explanation for this difference in mortality is probably the explanation also for another striking feature of the epidemic—the absence of a devastating diphtheria epidemic in Boston. This is one of the most difficult phases of the "throat distemper" to explain. The Boston epidemic of 1735-36 was scarlet fever and therefore not pertinent to this discussion. It will be recalled that between 1735 and 1740 the "Eastward Distemper" slowly advanced towards Boston and actually reached some of the surrounding towns—Marblehead, Malden, and Cambridge—but no evidence of any great diphtheria epidemic in Boston itself has come to light. Certainly there was ample contact with the "Eastward," for almost every New England diarist tells of frequent visits, and there are numerous records of whole families moving into the chief trade center of the colonies. It will also be recalled that some of the country towns lost from one-third to one-half of their children and if Boston had suffered to the same degree, three or four thousand children would have lost their lives. The people had ample reason to be fearful, but nothing like that occurred. What is the explanation? Those who believe that the "throat distemper" was an epidemic of a single disease might argue that the New Hampshire disease was scarlet fever and therefore one could not expect to find a second Boston epidemic, but I believe there is too much contemporary evidence against this view, and besides, even on these grounds one has to assume the presence of some immunity difference to explain the lower Boston death-rate. It might also be argued that my Boston facts and figures are incomplete and that Boston may have experienced a serious diphtheria epidemic. If that were true it would seem that William Douglass, ever on the alert for new and unusual diseases, would surely have left us an account. A few of his remarks can be construed as favoring diphtheria, but there is no ground for the belief that he saw more than sporadic cases. Moreover, I can find no evidence of diphtheria in Roxbury or Medford, towns near Boston, and even in Dorchester, Lynn, Salem, and Watertown, where there is some slight evidence of the disease, one can find no great epidemics comparable to the epidemics in the New Hampshire towns. It is possible that Boston and the larger surrounding towns escaped simply because they were on the fringe of the epidemic and we know that epidemics do have geographical limits although they are not so easy to explain. All in all, however, the most plausible reason for this absence of a large diphtheria epidemic in Boston is that there was a relative immunity as a result of the endemic presence of the disease before 1735. There are not many historical facts to support such an assumption, but John Walton's *Essay on the Rattles* (Boston, 1732) may be mentioned here. This essay, with its quaint theories of disease, though not written in Boston, can be taken as indirect evidence that diphtheria had been frequently observed in many New England towns, and perhaps, as the records are more thoroughly searched, some other more convincing evidence will be found. But it would be unwise to insist that a possible difference in immunity was the true explanation for the differences in mortality in the separate provinces until there are more substantial facts on the medical history of each town. In a complicated subject such as this, where population changes, diet, inheritance, and many other factors are involved, one must be content merely to offer theories and not attempt to offer proof.

— 3 —

Why a diphtheria epidemic occurred in Kingston in 1735, or what may have been the original cause of the "throat distemper," is another question not so easily answered. The early colonists had many explanations. The sick pig in Kingston, the default of ministers' salaries, the mortally infected air, Original Sin, dead caterpillars, God's Holy Anger, and various other causes were considered at different times, but because modern science is still uncertain about many things concerning epidemics, we cannot dismiss all their theories with a haughty smile. Even our latest theories are constantly being challenged by the accumulation of new facts and some of the science of today may easily become the quaint and ridiculous folk-lore of tomorrow.

Possible explanations again depend somewhat upon whether or not diphtheria had been prevalent in New Hampshire. The supposition that it was a new disease would correspond with the fact that no clinical evidence of the disease has been found, particularly in Kingston where the epidemic began, but that is not proof that diphtheria did not exist. At that time, however, there was a firm belief that "there never was ye like Before in this Country" and over and over again the opinion was everywhere expressed that it was a new disease. But diphtheria has frequently been described as a new disease in other, more recent, epidemics and so the popular contemporary opinion is no proof of scientific fact. Therefore, one cannot be certain that diphtheria was a new disease in Kingston and the other frontier towns; the most that can be said is that these towns had not previously experienced such a malignant epidemic.

On the other hand, there is some other indirect evidence that diphtheria was not a new disease in New Hampshire. As pointed out above, Dover, Exeter, Hampton, and Portsmouth, the four oldest towns, seemed to have fewer deaths in proportion to their populations than had the smaller outlying towns, and if this difference can be attributed to a difference in population immunity, then diphtheria was probably endemic in the oldest towns. Moreover, Fitch's figures reveal the very significant fact that ninety-six per cent of the deaths were among children under twenty years of age. This age distribution is similar to that found today with certain diseases such as whooping cough, chicken pox, and measles. These diseases do not attack children because of any special predilection for a particular age group, for when they occur on islands where there is little contact with the civilized world, all ages are attacked; and even in seventeenth century New England, when measles epidemics were infrequent, the disease attacked adults as well as children. However, in most populations where there is intimate social contact, these diseases attack only the children because the adults are immune, this immunity having been acquired as the result of earlier infection. But many adults are immune to diphtheria when there is no apparent history of previous infection and hence it has been assumed that these persons must have had subclinical or very mild infections of which they were unaware. Lately, however, the question has arisen whether or not diphtheria immunity is acquired solely by previous exposure to the disease. It has been found that the Eskimos are naturally immune without apparent prior contact,[193] and Jordan[194] has found that some animals approaching maturity show blood reactions which indicate that they acquire immunity against diseases to which, so far as is known, they have never been exposed. On this theory, Fitch's figures would be explained as a natural growth process, and independent of exposure to diphtheria. Nevertheless, the weight of opinion at the present time is that adult immunity to diphtheria results only from contact with diphtheria toxin and the conclusion seems warranted that, in spite of no history of diphtheria in Kingston, the disease must surely have been present in a mild form at least.[195]

Inasmuch as there is some difference of opinion, let it be merely supposed that diphtheria was actually unknown in Kingston, and that a malignant type was carried in from some other infected town. Perhaps some travelling "pedalar," visiting relative or friend, or perhaps some one of the families that moved into town and entered intimately into church and social life, served as a carrier of the disease. We are certain that most of the Kingston children had no immunity. The powder was dry and only a spark was needed for an explosion.

This theory adequately explains the Kingston facts and also the subsequent spread throughout New Hampshire. The time element in the progress of the epidemic is compatible with the supposition that each town received its initial infection from a neighboring town or from Kingston, the original source. Indeed, if all the facts were

---

[193] Literature quoted by P. H. Harmon. *Amer. J. Dis. Children.* 1934, June, p. 1224.

[194] E. O. Jordan. *Proc. Exper. Biol. & Med.*, xxx, 446.

[195] There were about fifteen or twenty deaths among children in the autumn and early winter of 1730, with about two to six deaths each month. Two of Jedidiah Philbrick's children died in September; two of Thomas Dent's children died in December; there were no other multiple deaths. These findings are compatible with a mild diphtheria but could also be explained on the basis of a dysentery or smallpox epidemic. There are no available clinical descriptions.

known, especially about contacts with healthy carriers, this theory might explain the spread to Maine and Massachusetts. But it does not explain the origin of a similar epidemic at nearly the same time in the Newark Mountains of New Jersey, for it does not seem likely that the two epidemics arose from a single source. At that time, overland travel was difficult; there was only one regular coach

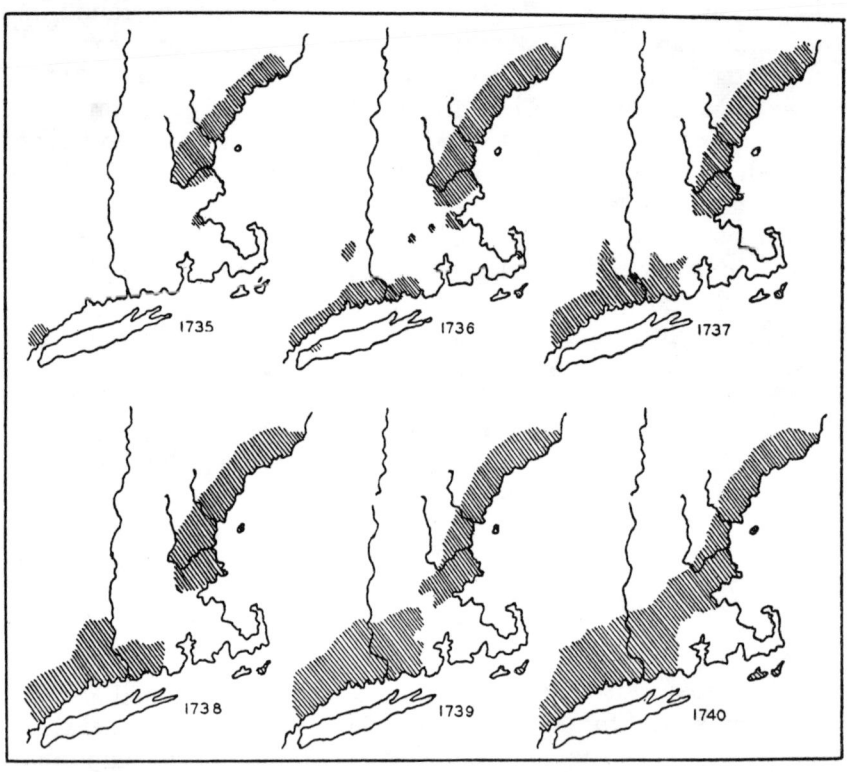

The progressive spread of the epidemic during the years 1735 to 1740 from the two foci, one in Connecticut, the other in New Hampshire.

between Boston and New York, and most long trips were made by water. If the two epidemics had first appeared in seaport towns, some direct relation might be suspected, but, as it happened, both began in isolated inland towns. There was considerable migration from New Hampshire and Connecticut to New Jersey but the disease appeared in New Jersey first. Therefore, it is probable that the two epidemics were independent. Furthermore, there is some evidence, as yet unconfirmed, of a similar malignant diphtheria epidemic occurring in the West Indies at the same time that the "throat distemper" appeared in New England.[196] So the various epidemics are not easily explained on the assumption that the disease was carried from previously infected areas unless an unusual coincidence is assumed.

Thus, we are led to consider the possibility that diphtheria was already present in Kingston and in New Jersey and that during the spring of 1735, and for some unexplained reason, the organism suddenly underwent some change and took on an added virulence and infectivity. This theory finds some support in our experience with other epidemics and is related to the so-called cyclic variation in virulence of diseases. Smallpox today is supposed to be milder than was the smallpox of the eighteenth century, and scarlet fever, influenza, and measles are thought to vary in virulence from time to time. By far the best evidence that diphtheria became more virulent about 1735 is found in the *Vital Records* of almost every New Hampshire and Massachusetts town. At that period one can find hundreds of instances of multiple deaths, whereas, before then, multiple deaths were very infrequent and most of those that have been found can be accounted for by dysentery and smallpox. This sudden increase in multiple deaths is so striking that I have used it as evidence of the "throat distemper" in some few towns where other records could not be found. That it was a new and unusual experience for the colonists is also shown by that notice in the *New York Gazette* which said that the burial of four Boynton children in one grave was an event "seldom known in this part of the world." We can understand how the colonists may have failed to mention sporadic cases of diphtheria and how they may have confused various types of disease, but a disease that frequently killed from three to eight children in a family within about a month was not likely to be quickly forgotten. And so it seems that this sudden marked increase in the occurrence of multiple deaths can be taken as evidence of an increased virulence in diphtheria which, if true, would be a reasonable explanation for the epidemic. The only experimental evidence bearing on this point, however, seems to contradict this conception of the cause of an epidemic. Webster,[197] while studying experimentally produced epidemics among mice, could

---
[196] William Douglass: *Practical History* . . . p. 13. *Boston Weekly Post Boy*, Aug. 30, 1736.
[197] L. T. Webster: loc. cit.

find no evidence that an organism varies in virulence before, during, or after an epidemic, and his results seem to show that explosive epidemic outbreaks may result from changes in dosage of the organism or from changes connected with the host. Therefore, however apparent the increased virulence of diphtheria during 1735 may seem, we cannot be certain of such a simple explanation.

Another possibility to be considered is suggested by other results in experimental epidemiology. It has been found that among groups of mice that were previously infected with certain organisms, recurrent epidemic waves could be produced merely by adding susceptible mice to the infected community at a constant rate.[198] The epidemics which occurred when the proportion of immigrants reached a certain level were very similar to natural epidemics. Now, if it is supposed that diphtheria was present in New Hampshire before 1735, the conditions are somewhat analogous to those in the experiments with mice. Perhaps it was merely coincidental, nevertheless, the New England and New Jersey epidemics happened to occur immediately following the start of a rapid growth in population. This relation as it concerns New Hampshire is illustrated in the graph and similar graphs could be drawn for the other colonies. Moreover, this was a period of land speculation and the population increases naturally occurred in frontier towns where land was more easily obtained. Perhaps by 1735 this population increase was just enough to upset the balance between immunized and unimmunized subjects and an epidemic was the result. The populations of the other provinces were also rapidly increasing at the same time and therefore the apparently

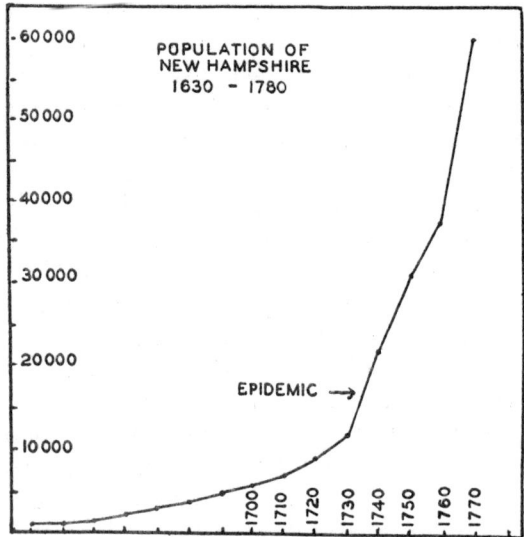

The relation of the occurrence of the epidemic to the growth in population. Compiled from statistics in *American Dictionary of Dates*, by C. L. Damon. Boston, 1921, vol. 1.

---

[198] Greenwood and Topley: Quoted by Webster.

independent but simultaneous diphtheria epidemics can possibly be explained.

This conception of the outbreak of diphtheria finds additional support in the circumstances surrounding some other epidemics. If the development of the New England frontier was attended by epidemics of diphtheria it would be interesting to know if the development of other American frontiers was also attended by similar epidemics. I cannot offer very much scientific evidence, but it is probably more than a coincidence that such epidemics did actually occur when the American frontier was extended beyond the Alleghanies. In Drake's account of *The Principal Diseases of the Interior Valley of North America*[199] we find descriptions of epidemics among the first settlers of Kentucky and Ohio in 1791 and 1793; and in Paris, Kentucky (1821), St. Clairsville, Ohio (1833), Greene County, Ohio (1838-40), and St. Louis (1845), there were severe epidemics of "malignant sore throat" which were very similar indeed, even to the very high mortality and the frequency of multiple deaths, to the "throat distemper" of New England in 1735. But here again, our facts are too few to warrant definite conclusions and we must leave a very interesting subject with merely theoretical explanations.

---

[199] Daniel Drake: *A Systematic Treatise*. Phila., 1854, pp. 594-95.

OBSERVATIONS
On that terrible 𝔇𝔦𝔰𝔢𝔞𝔰𝔢

Vulgarly called

The *Throat-Distemper.*

WITH

Advices as to the

Method of Cure.

In a Letter to a Friend.

By J. DICKINSON, A.M.

BOSTON: Printed and Sold by S. KNEELAND and T. GREEN, in Queenstreet, over against the Prison. 1740.

To the READER.

THE Reverend Mr Dickinson, when at Boston nigh two Years since, being consulted by several Gentlemen (anxious for themselves and others) about a most malignant Disease, which had raged for a long Time in the Place where he lives, and which had commenc'd its fatal Progress in these Parts, was desir'd to draw up his Observations in writing, with a View to printing the same for the publick Benefit. Upon that Occasion he wrote the following Letter: which now that we have a fresh Alarm by a Return of that astonishing Distemper among us, it's thought a proper Season to publish it for a common Good.

 Several of our ablest Physicians, upon the perusal of it, have express'd their Satisfaction in the Author's Account of the various Phænomena of the Malady and his Method of Cure —— His Observations are the Result of a long Series of Practice and Experience, and seem founded in the exactest Judgment. His Informations are as full and particular, as any we've seen, and studiously deliver'd in the easiest Language, to accommodate unlearned Readers. —— The surprizing Mortality of this Distemper is enough to attract every one's serious Attention; and in such an extraordinary Case every compassionate Friend to Mankind, will be ready to impart any useful Reflections: Which is a sufficient Apology both for the Author and the Publisher.

Cambridge, Aug. 5.
  1 7 4 0.

A LETTER, &c.

SIR,

IN Compliance with your Desire, I shall now communicate to you some of those Observations I have made upon that extraordinary Disease, which has made such awful Desolations in the Country, commonly called *the Throat-Distemper*.

This Distemper first began in these Parts, in *Febr.* 1734,5 The long Continuance and universal Spread of it among us, has given me abundant Opportunity to be acquainted with it in all its Forms.

The first Assault was in a Family about ten Miles from me, which proved fatal to eight of the Children in about a Fortnight. Being called to visit the distressed Family, I found upon my arrival there, one of the Children newly dead, which gave me the Advantage of a *Dissection*, and thereby a better Acquaintance with the Nature of the Disease, than I could otherwise have had: From which (and other like) Observations, I came pretty

pretty early into the Methods of Cure that I have not yet seen Reason to change.

There have few Distempers been ever known, that have put on a greater *variety of Types*, and appear'd with more different Symptoms, than this has done; which makes it necessary to be something particular in describing it, in order to set it in a just View, and to propose the Methods of Cure necessary in its several Appearances. And

1. I take this Disease to be naturally an *Eruptive milliary Fever*: and when it appears as such, it usually begins with a Shivering, a Chill, or with Stretching, or Yawning; which is quickly succeeded with a sore Throat, a Tumefaction of the Tonsils, Uvula and Epiglottis, and sometimes of the Jaws, and even of the whole Throat & Neck. The Fever is often acute, the Pulse quick & high, and the Countenance florid. The Tonsils first, and in a little Time the whole Throat covered with a whitish Crustula, the Tongue furr'd, and the Breath fetid. Upon the 2d, 3d, or 4th Day, if proper Methods are used, the Patient is cover'd with a milliary Eruption, in some exactly resembling the *Measles*, in others more like the *Scarlet Fever* (for which Distemper it has frequently been mistaken) but in others it very much resembles the confluent *Small Pox*. When the Eruption is finished, the Tumefaction every where subsides, the Fever abates, and the Slough in the Throat casts off and fal's. The Eruption often disappears about the 6th or 7th Day; tho' it sometimes continues visible much longer. After the Eruption is over, the Cuticle scales and falls off, as in the Conclusion of the Scarlet Fever. If after the

the Crife of this Difeafe Purging be neglected, the Sick may feem to recover Health & Strength for a while; yet they frequently in a little Time fall again into grievous Diforders; fuch as a great proftration of Strength, lofs of Appetite, hectical Appearances, fometimes great Dimnefs of Sight, and often fuch a weaknefs in the Joints as deprives them of the Ufe of all their Limbs; and fome of them are affected with fcorbutick Symptoms of almoft every Kind.

When this Diftemper appears in the Form now defcribed, it is not very dangerous: I have feldom feen any die with it, unlefs by a fudden Loofenefs, that calls in the Eruptions; or by fome very irregular Treatment. But there are feveral other very different Appearances of the Difeafe, which are attended with more frightful & deadly Confequences.

2. It frequently begins with a flight Indifpofition, much refembling an ordinary *Cold*, with a liftlefs Habit, a flow & fcarce difcernible Fever, fome forenefs of the Throat and Tumefaction of the Tonfils; and perhaps a running of the Nofe, the Countenance pale, and the Eyes dull and heavy. The Patient is not confin'd, nor any Danger apprehended for fome Days, till the Fever gradually increafes, the whole Throat, and fometimes the Roof of the Mouth and Noftrils, are covered with a *cankerous Cruft*, which corrodes the contiguous Parts, and frequently terminates in a mortal Gangreen, if not by feafonable Applications prevented. The *Stomach* is fometimes, and the *Lungs* often, covered with the fame *Cruftula*. The *former* Cafe is difcovered

ed by a vehement Sickness of the Stomach, a perpetual vomiting; and sometimes by ejecting of black or rusty and fetid Matter, having Scales like Bran mixed with it, which is a certain Index of a *fatal Mortification.* ---- When the *Lungs* are thus affected, the Patient is first afflicted with a dry hollow Cough, which is quickly succeeded with an extraordinary Hoarseness and total Loss of the Voice, with the most distressing asthmatick Symptoms and difficulty of Breathing, under which the poor miserable Creature struggles, until released by a perfect *Suffocation,* or stoppage of Breath.——This *last* has been the fatal Symptom, under which the most have sunk, that have died in these Parts. And indeed there have comparatively but few recovered, whose Lungs have been thus affected. All that I have seen to get over this dreadful Symptom, have fallen into a *Ptyalism* or Salivation, equal to a *petit Flux de Bouche,* and have by their perpetual Cough expectorated incredible Quantities of a tough whitish Slough from their Lungs, for a considerable Time together. And on the other Hand, I have seen large Pieces of this Crust, several Inches long and near an Inch broad, torn from the Lungs by the vehemence of the Cough, without any Signs of Digestion, or possibility of obtaining it.

Before I dismiss this Head, I must observe, that the *Fever* which introduces the terrible Symptoms now described, does not always make such a slow and gradual Approach: but sometimes makes a fiercer Attack; and might probably be thrown off by the Eruptions, and this
Train

Train of Terrors prevented, if proper Methods were seasonably used.

3. This Distemper sometimes appears in the Form of an *Erysipelas*. The Face suddenly inflames and swells, the Skin appears of a darkish Red, the Eyes are closed with the Tumefaction, which also sometimes extends through the whole Neck and Chest. Blisters or other small Ulcers here and there break out upon the Tumor, which corrode the adjacent Parts; and quickly bring on a Mortification, if not by some happy Means prevented. Some that are thus affected, are at the same Time exercised with all the terrible *internal* Symptoms above described; and some with none of them. If this inflamed Tumor be not quickly discussed, it will (I think) always prove mortal.

4. Another Appearance of this Disease is in external *Ulcers*: which break out frequently behind the Ears; sometimes they cover the whole Head and Forehead; sometimes they appear in the Arm-Pits, Groins, Navil, Buttocks or Seat; and sometimes in any of the extream Parts. These are covered with the same Kind of whitish *Crustula*, above described, which also corrodes the contiguous Parts; and quickly, if not prevented, ends in a *Mortification*. I have ordinarily observed, that if these outward Ulcers are speedily cured, the Throat and internal Parts remain free from the abovementioned terrible Symptoms; otherwise the miserable Patient must pass thro' the whole tragical Scene of Terrors before represented, if an external Gangreen don't terminate his Agony and Life together.

5. Sometimes

5. Sometimes this Disease appears first in *Bubo's* under the Ears, Jaws, or Chin, or in the Arm-Pits, or Groin. These, if quickly ripened, make a considerable Discharge ; which brings a salutary End to the Disease ; otherwise they quickly end in a fatal Mortification ; or else bring on the whole foremention'd Tragedy.

6. This Disease appears sometimes in the Form of a *Quinsey*. The Lungs are inflamed, the Throat and especially the Epiglottis exceedingly tumefied. In a few Hours the Sick is brought to the Height of an *Orthopnœa* ; and cannot breathe but in an erect Posture, and then with great Difficulty and Noise. This may be distinguished from an *Angina*, by the *Crustula* in the Throat, which determines it to be a Sprout from the same Root with the Symptoms described above. In this Case the Patient sometimes dies in twenty four Hours. I have not seen any one survive the third Day. But thro' the divine Goodness these Symptoms have been more rarely seen among *us*, and there have been but few in this Manner snatch'd out of the World.

As the Symptoms of this Distemper are very different, so the *Methods of Cure* should be respectively accommodated to them ; and I shall therefore consider them distinctly.

When this Distemper makes its Attack with the Symptoms of a *high Fever*, a *florid* Countenance &c. (as in the *first* Case described) the *first Intention*, to be pursued towards a Cure, is to bring out the *Eruptions* as soon as possible ; to which End, I order the Patient to be confin'd in
Bed,

Bed, and put into a gentle breathing *Sweat*, till they appear. A *Tea* made with Virginian *Snake-Root* and English *Saffron*, with a few Grains of *Cochineal*; A *Posset* made with *Carduus Mariæ* boil'd in Milk, and turn'd with Wine, the *Lapis contrayerva*, or *Gascoign-Powder*; any or all of these, as Occasions requires, answer to this Purpose, and seldom fail of Success.

One of the most dangerous Circumstances that attend this Disease, is a *Looseness*, that frequently happens upon the first Appearance of the Eruptions; which must be speedily restrain'd, and the Belly kept bound, lest the morbifick Matter, evaporated by the Pores, be recalled into the Blood, and prove suddenly fatal.——— To that Purpose, I ordinarily advise to *Venice-Treacle*, or liquid *Laudanum*, which commonly answer all Intentions. But if the Patient should be in a *dozing* Habit, that these cannot be used, or if these should fail of Success, any other *Astringent* may be used that is proper in a *Diarrhœa*.

The *Ulcers* in the Throat should be constantly cleansed, from the Time of their first Appearance. I have found the following Method most successful to this Purpose. *Take* Roman Vitriol, *let it lie as near the Fire as a Man can bear his Hand, till it be thoroughly calcined and turn'd white*: Put about eight Grains *of this into half a Pint of Water*: Lay *down the Tongue with a* Spatula; *and gently wash off as much of the Crust as will easily separate, with a fine Ragg fastned to the End of a Probe, or Stick, and wet in this Liquor made warm.* This Operation should be repeated every three or four Hours.

After the Eruptions are quite gone, the Patient should be *purged* two or three Times, to prevent the Consequences above described; and this Rule should be observed in every Form of the Disease.

If after the Crise of this Disease, in any of its Appearances, the Sick should fall into any of the Disorders mentioned under the first Head, such as Loss of Strength, a feverish Habit, Dimness of Sight, Weakness of the Joynts &c. *Repeated Purging*, as far as the Patient's Strength will bear, with *Elixir Propretatis* given twice a Day in a Glass of generous Wine, will constantly remove these Difficulties.

When this Disease makes a more slow and leisurely approach with a *lingering* Fever, *pale* Countenance &c. as described in the *second* Case; all Attempts to bring out the milliary Eruptions seem in vain. And therefore, tho' the Sick may be very much relieved by the *diaphoretick* Medicines abovementioned, if repeatedly used during the Course of the Illness; yet these are not to be depended upon for a Cure. But a brisk *Purge* should be also directed every third Day, and those Catharticks that are mixt with *Colomel* or *Mercurius dulcis*, are most likely to be serviceable, where the Age and Strength of the Patient will bear it.

If there be an extream *nauseating*, and vehement Sickness of the Stomach, that can't be otherwise quieted, an *Emetick* seems necessary; tho' I have not found Encouragement to use vomiting Physick in any other Case.

The *internal Ulcers* of the Throat should be treated as above directed; but if there be a great
Tume-

Tumefaction of the Glands, I order externally a Plaister of *Diachylon cum Gummi* and *de Ranis cum Mercurio* mixt; and internally the following Fumigation. *Take Wormwood, Penny-royal, the Tips of St. John's Wort, Camomile-Flowers and Elder-Flowers, of each equal Parts; boil very strong in Water; when boil'd, add as much Brandy or Rum as of this Decoction; steam the Throat thro' a Tunnel, as hot as can be born, three or four Times a Day.*

When the *Lungs* are seized with this cankerous *Crustula*, which is indicated by the Cough and Hoarseness above described, *Mercurial Catharticks* frequently repeated, seem the best of any Thing to promote Expectoration. I have also found Success in the Use of the Syrup of red Poppies and *Sperma Ceti* mixt.

When this Distemper appears in the Form of an *Erysipelas*, I have used the following Fomentation with good Success. *Take Wormwood, Mint, Elder-Flowers, Camomile-Flowers, the Tips of St. John's Wort, Fennel-Seeds pounded, and the lesser Centaury, equal Parts: Infuse in good Brandy or Jamaica Rum, in a Stone-Jugg well stop'd, and kept hot by the Fire: wet a Flannel Cloth with this; and after moderately squeezing out the Liquor, apply three or four double to the Tumor, as hot as can be born, every Hour.* — In this Case I repeat *Purging*, as above directed.

As for the *external Ulcers* above described (under the 4th Head) they may be always safely and speedily cured, by applying once or twice a Day a good thick Pledget of fine Tow dipt in the above described *vitriolick Water.* I have never known this fail in a single Instance, when seasonably used. But then it must be observed, that some of these Ulcers will require this Water much sharper with the Vitriol, than others will bear. It should be so sharp as to bring off the Slough, dry up the flow of corrosive Humours, and promote a Digestion: but it must not be made a painful Caustick. In this the Practitioner's Discretion will guide him.

I need not say any more respecting the *Bubo's*, mentioned under the *fifth* Head; but that they must by all possible Means be ripen'd as quick as they can; and launced as soon as they are digested and found to contain any *Pus*.

I have not yet found any effectual Remedy in the 6th and last Case described.

Upon the Disease in *general*, I have made the following *Remarks*; which perhaps may be of some Use.

I have observ'd, that the *more acute* the *Fever* is on the first Seizure, the *less dangerous*; because there's more Hope of bringing out the Eruptions.

I have observ'd, that there's more Danger of receiving Injury from a *cold Air* in this, than in any eruptive Fever I have seen. The *Eruptions* are *easily struck in*; and therefore there ought to be all possible Care, that the Sick be not at all exposed to the Air, till the Eruptions are quite over and gone.

I have also observ'd, that there's much greater Danger from this Disease in *cold Weather*, than in hot. In cold Weather it most commonly appears in the Form described under the *second* Head;

while

while on the contrary, a hot Season very much forwards the Eruptions.

I have frequently obferv'd, that *once* having this Disease is no Security against a *second Attack*. I have known the same Person to have it *four Times* in one Year; the last of which prov'd mortal. I have known Numbers, that have passed thro' it in the *eruptive* Form in the *Summer* Season, that have died with it the succeeding *Fall* or *Winter*: tho' I have never seen any upon whom the *Eruptions* could be *brought out* more than *once*.

I have ordinarily obferv'd, that those who die with this Disease, have many *Purple-Spots* about them; which shews the Height of Malignity and Pestilential Quality in this terrible Distemper.

Thus, SIR, I have endeavour'd in the most plain and familiar Manner to answer your Demands. I have not attempted a *Philosophical* Inquiry into the Nature of this Disease, nor a *Rationale* upon the Methods of Cure. I have meant no more than briefly to communicate to you some of my *Experiences* in this Distemper, which I presume is all you expect from me. If this proves of any Service, I shall have Cause of Thankfulness: If not, you'll kindly accept my willingness to serve you, and to contribute what I can towards the Relief of the afflicted and miserable.

I am, SIR,

Elizabeth Town, N. Jersey
Febr. 20. 1738,9.

Your most humble Servant,

Jonathan Dickinson.

POSTSCRIPT.

SINCE I wrote this Letter, I am inform'd by a Gentleman of the Profession, who has had very great Improvement in this Distemper, That he has found out a *Method of Cure*, which seldom fails of Success in all the Forms of this Disease herein described, (the *first, fourth*, and *fifth* only excepted, which should be treated as above directed) and that is a *Decoction of the Root of the* Dart Weed, or (*as it is here called*) *the* Squaw-Root. *He orders about an* Ounce *of this Root to be boiled in a Quart of Water, to which he adds when strain'd, a Jill of* Rum *and two Ounces of* Loaf-Sugar; *and boils again to the Consumption of one quarter Part.* This he gives his Patients frequently to drink, and with this orders them frequently to gargle their Throats; allowing *no internal Medicine but this only*, during the whole Course of the Disease, excepting a *Purge* or two in the Conclusion. I have seen a surprizing Effect of this Method in one Instance; and shall make what further Observations I can: And if this answers my present Hopes, I shall endeavour to give you further Information.

The *Dart-Weed* grows with a strait Stalk six or eight Foot high, is jointed every eight or ten Inches apart; and bears a large white Tassel on the Top, when in the Flower. The Root is black and bitterish.

F I N I S.

Practical HISTORY

OF

A New Epidemical Eruptive Miliary Fever, with an Angina Ulcusculosa

Which

Prevailed in *Boston* New-England in the Years 1735 and 1736.

By *William Douglass*, M. D.

BOSTON, N.E.

Printed and sold by *Thomas Fleet*, at the Sign of the *Heart* and *Crown* in Cornhill. 1736.

TO

A Medical Society

in *Boston*.

Gentlemen,

THIS Piece of Medical History does naturally address it self to you, considering that I have the pleasure of being one of your number, that you have been fellow labourers in the management of this distemper, and therefore competent judges of this performance, and that where difficult or extraordinary Cases have occurred in any of your private practice, I was favoured to visit the Patients in order to make a minute clinical enquiry: in short, without your assistance this piece would have been less perfect, and not so well vouched.

As this distemper continues to spread and prevail in several Towns of this and the neighbouring Provinces, I thought it might prove a piece of humanity and benevolence, if after many months diligent observations made in most of the varieties which occur in this Illness, I did endeavour to reduce them to some easy distinct Historical and Practical Method. The vanity of appearing as an Author or writer was no inducement, because we all know that in a plantation life neither honour nor credit are to be acquired by writing. It is not published by way *of a Quack bill to procure Patients and their money, as has been the practice of some void of modesty and truth; because the Distemper is almost over in* Boston, *and while it prevailed here I could not well have attended more patients than what I had from time to time under my care, and make with attention the proper observations at the same time.*

A secondary reason for my writing is, to induce some Gentlemen of the profession in our other Provinces and Colonies, where this distemper does or may prevail; to give some account of its appearance with them, in order to discover what influence, progress of time, varieties of climate and Soil may have in the phænomina of this disease. This method, of taking things originally that is from the life, if pursued (but by abler hands) in the Epidemical Distempers which may from time to time happen amongst us, may be of considerable advantage in Physick.

A Speculation that is a novelle might have been composed sooner, but not a real History: for as amongst Naturalists, many repeated observations and experiments are requisite to form established truths or conclusions; so it ought certainly to be in the practice of Medicine, where no affair of Speculation or curiosity, but the life and death of a fellow Citizen is the object of our enquiry.

Yours, &c.

William Douglass.

The Practical History of a new Epidemical *Miliary Fever* with an *Angina Ulcusculosa.*

THIS Distemper did emerge 20·h. *May*, 1735. in *Kingston* Township 50 Miles Eastward from *Boston*; it was no foreign importation, *Kingston* being an inland place, of no Trade or considerable communication. The first seized was a *child who died in three Days Illness*; about a Week thereafter in another Family at four Miles distance, three Children were seized successively, and died also the third Day; it continues spreading gradually in that Township, seizing here and there particular Families with that degree of violence, that *of the first circiter forty decumbents none recovered* as we were informed. It was vulgarly called the *Throat Illness*, or *a Plague in the Throat*, and alarmed the Provinces of *New-England* very much. Some died of a sudden or acute *Necrosis*; but most of them by a *Symptomatick affection of the Fauces or Neck*; that is by *Sphacelations* or corrosive *Ulcerations* in the *Fauces*, or by *an infiltration and tumefaction* in the Chops and fore part of the Neck, so turged, as to bring all upon a level between the chin and *sternum*, occasioning a *strangulation* of the Patient in a very short time.

After a few Weeks it spreads into the neighbouring Townships, but with more mildness. The first *appearance* that we can recollect of it in *Boston*, was 20th *August* in a Child of Capt. *Stannys* at the North End; having *white specks* in the Throat, and a *cutaneous efflorescence:* A few more in the same Neighbourhood were seized in like manner, about the same time. Towards the end of *September* it appeared in several parts of the Town, with a complaint of *soreness in the Throat, Tonsils swelled and speckt, Uvula relaxed, slight Fever, flush in the Face, and an Erysipelas like efflorescence on the neck, chest and extremities;* but being of no fatal or bad consequence, nothing more than a common cold was suspected. Our first alarm was from a young Man *How* Æt. 20. in the beginning of *October*: His *History* runs thus; He was lately arrived from *Exeter* to the Eastward, where his Brother died of this Illness; his *Symptoms* were great prostration of Strength, a speck in one of the *Tonsils*, colliquative *Sweats, Pulse* not high and full, but low, hard, stringy, unequal and more frequent than natural, *deglutition* good to the last, no *Sphacelation* in the Throat, no eruption; from a rash inconsiderate opinion of forcibly quelling the *Malignity*, he was thrice let Blood, had some Emeticks and Catharticks adminstred, and *by profuse evacuations was gradually reduced, so as to die of a gentle decay of natural Strength*, the 6th Day of Illness.

Beginning of *November* it spread considerably in *Boston*, especially amongst *Children*, with more violent Symptoms, and severals die of it in various Periods: it seemed to be at the hight, as to Numbers ailing and quantity of Deaths, the second Week of *March*; that Week there were 24 Burials, whereas *communibus annis* in that Season they are only 9 or 10 *per* Week.

It

It is generally in so considerable a Degree *more favourable in Boston*, than in the Townships where it first prevailed; that many can scarce be persuaded of its being the same Distemper: It is nevertheless essentially the same, there is no Symptom, even the most malignant that has appeared in *New Hampshire*, but what the like has occured in *Boston.* Perhaps *Boston* dry healthy air, good feeding, constitutions less *Psorick*, and the better management of the Sick, favoured us; the reasons for its proving more mortal in the other Towns, may be, the Country woodland and fresh water damps, (the *Sheep* in fenny lands are most susceptible of and suffer most by the *Rot*) their coarse Food, salt Pork diet, *Psorick* Constitutions, (which is one of the principal *Endemial distemperatures in New-England*) bad Lodgings, and that *mischievous Practice* of using this Distemper with profuse evacuations, whereby the laudable and salutary *cuticular* eruption has been so perverted as to be noticeable only in a few, and in these it was called a *Scarlet Fever*; the great prostration of Strength essential to this Distemper is so much increased, as to render *Nature* an under match for the assaults of this Illness and its consequences. In fact to the Eastward in some Country Towns, at certain times have died 1 in 3 of the Sick, in others 1 in 4, in scarce any fewer than 1 in 6, whereas in *Boston* not above 1 in 35 have died.

As in most *Epidemical* acute Illnesses, especially *eruptive Fevers*, (witness the *Small Pox*) so in this, are very many varities or degrees, from the most gentle and *benign* to the most *malignant*. Symptoms did vary chiefly from something inscrutable in the *Constitutions* of Families and Persons; the *Scropholous and Psorick* were the most susceptible of it, and
did

did suffer most by it; the *Regimen* had a considerable influence, here some who might have survived the *natural Symptoms* did succumb by profuse U. S. and other evacuations, one of the most essential Symptoms of this Distemper (as before hinted) being *great prostration of Strength*. In so great variety it is not possible to give any concise *scholastick* description, which may comprehend all: We shall therefore, as a *Standard* first describe the most frequent sort, as it appeared in good constitutions.

A previous *listlesness* and languishing countenance for a Day or two, or some other *prænuncia* as u. g. wet Nurses loosing their Milk. The first attack is somewhat of a *chill* or shivering; soon after follows *Head ake* or some other versatile *spasmodick pains*, as pain in the back, joints, side, *&c*; a vomiting or *nausea*, or in some constitutions which are not easily provoked to vomit, only a certain uneasiness or sickness at Stomach; at the same time the *Uvula* but chiefly the *Tonsils* were tumified, inflamed and painful, with some white *specks*; then follows a flush in the Face and some *miliary eruptions* there, with a benign *mild Fever*, the same efflorescence soon after appears on the neck, chest and extremities; the 3d or 4th Day, Eruption is at the hight and well defined with fair intervals; the flushing goes off gradually, with a general *itching*; and in a Day or two more the *cuticle* scales or peels off, especially in the extremities: At the same time the cream coloured sloughs or specks in the *Fauces* become loose and cast off, and tumefactions there do subside. The Tongue from the beginning is fur'd as in a *Mercurial ptyalism*, urine high coloured, Blood by U. S. more *florid* than natural, in the whole course of the Distemper a very *great prostration*

tion of Strength, and faintness upon recovery, *nervous pains* and weakness in the joints, particularly in the neck, wrists and ancles; universal tenderness to the touch; a tickling guttural cough, some short *Hectick flushings*, and loss of *en bon point*. As in the Measles there is a peculiar smell, so in our Distemper the *effluvia* from the Patient have a proper smell; in Children as if troubled with *Worms*, in grown Persons the *rancid smell* of foul Bed Linnen. The *alvine excrement* is of a dark cast and very fetid.

This Standard kind when left to nature, with a warm soft *Regimen*, had generally an easy and salutary course in six or seven Days; but when by a hot cordial method, or on the other extreme, by being too much exposed to the cold, or by officious *profuse evacuations* Nature was disturbed in her Work; the Distemper was protracted, or some consequential ails from an imperfect defecation ensued.

Where Nature required any assistance, the principal *intentions* were with regard to the cuticular eruption and the *ulcuscula* in the Throat. Any Affection of the Throat does frequently produce a natural *ptyalism*: *Mercurials* used with discretion are a kind of specifick in such like ulcers & *ulcuscula*, and in fact here they moistned the Throat and Mouth, stopt the spreading of the *ulcuscula*, and promoted the casting off of the sloughs; and as an accessory advantage (the Patients being mostly Children) *destroy'd Worms*: amongst all its preparations *Calomel* answered best, the gentle vomiting or few stools that it occasioned in some, did not confound the natural course of the Distemper; *Turbith* proves generally too strong a revulsion, and the Eruption is thereby too much diverted; this

Distemper did not well bear any other evacuations but *Mercurials*. Any detergent *Gargle*, with an addition of the *Tincture of Myrrh and Aloes*, was of good use, especially for the *Ulcuscula*, and did promote the discharge of a ropy Phlegm lodged in the *Fauces*. As to the *cuticular efflorescence*, it was not a scarlet *suffusion*, but a *miliary* palpable eruption, or in lieu thereof in some constitutions a continued gentle breathing *Sweat*; and in a very few, who have naturally a *liberior transitus* by the *Pores* than is usual, no sensible cuticular excretion; in all the morbid *effluvia* discovered themselves by their peculiar smell: These were with good effect sollicited by *Snake-root Tea*; or (as in some Persons) where this did occasion an *ardor* or burning heat, instead of a breathing mellow Sweat, *Sp. C. C.* or any other volatile Spirit in small Herb Teas answered well. *Blisters* and *Suppedanea*, in the beginning where Symptoms were not violent, occasioned a protracted Eruption; in some immediately upon their application, the Eruptions vanished or became less vivid. When the Eruption began to decline a few *loose Stools* were very refreshing. The Patient being up, and having recovered a competent degree of Strength, is *to be purged* once or twice, to carry off any feculency that may have remained in the Blood and Juices.

For a more distinct conception of the *varieties in this Distemper*, they may be reduced to three *Classes*.

I Those who die the first, second and third day of Illness, by an irremediable *Necrosis of the Oeconomy*: in such the Seizure is generally sudden, a sinking pain at the Stomach, an extreme prostration of Strength, a titubating low pulse, in some a stupor, in others a delirium, in some children con-

convulsions, and all of them generally die dozie: they are attended with some *colliquation*, as continued vomiting, purging, profuse Sweats, bloatedness of the habit, an infiltration like that of the *Mumps* vulgarly so called, one or more of these: in general the texture of their blood and juices is much destroy'd and rendred an incoherent puddle of corruption; in fact immediately upon (sometimes before) their *exit*, they have an intolerable *fœtor*. In this Class U. S. and other evacuations did accelerate death.

II. Those where the distemper has its common or ordinary course; here the 6 or 7 day seems to be *critical*, and the Symptoms of death or recovery do generally then begin to manifest themselves. Some by peculiarity of constitution, and from improper administrations do die or have an incipicent recovery sooner: others for the like reasons or some particular accidents (u. g. if about the time of regular *menstruation*, the complicated fret occasions worse Symtoms, and of longer continuance) have this period protracted and in such (where death is inevitable) the Symptoms of death may continue a day or two longer, that is the Patient may die the eighth or ninth day. All who continue ill after that period, belong to the third Class, that is of consequential ails.

The Symtoms of *bad Omen* in this Class, are very great prostration of strength, dejection and despondency of mind, titubating low pulse, incessant vomitings purgings or sweats, Tonsils much inflamed endangering strangulation, the specks in the *Fauces* of a brownish or leaden colour, or ragged and jagged, a continued *jactantia* in some, in others *a stupor*, refusal of *assumenda* even of diluting common

mon drinks, a dry parched skin, Eruptions appearing and difappearing alternately, Eruption univerfal of a dark redifh caft continuing *crude* many days (becaufe in this as in all eruptive Fevers, the darker or more livid the efflorefcence, the more malignant) where the *miliary* puftles are large, diftinct and pale like a *chryftaline Small-Pox*; where ftrong Cordials and *Alexipharmicks* have been ufed, the face, eye-lids, arms, hands, legs, feet fwell, and are of a dark red complexion, as in the moft malignant Small-Pox; in children if the *velum Palati* be much affected, with an *ichorous* difcharge by the Nofe; where many *mucous* linings are expectorated, refembling the cuticle raifed by Vefications; when *pus* was brought up, where no floughs or exulcerations could be feen in the *Fauces*; where without any difficulty in fwallowing, this affection has reached down the *Bronchia* unto the Lungs with the Symptoms of a *New-England Quinfey*, and was erronioufly deemed fuch: the deeper in the *Thorax* the complaint the greater the danger: in fome young children with fcarce any appearance in the Throat, fpreading Ulcers did form behind the Ears in the place where Infants have a natural Iffue or running. In fome the Tongue did throw off a flough or *Exuvia*, retaining the impreffions of the Papillæ; being a *Mucus* infpiffated, and of the fame nature with thofe mucous linings expectorated from the *Bronchia* or *Oefophagus*. Some have had impoftumations in the *Fauces*, with a fatal ftrangulation, while others have efcaped by the difcharge of *Ichorous* curdly matter. Some efpecially of the adult female kind, have had *Hyfterical* or Nervous Suffocations; but of no bad confequence, unlefs officioufly and ignorantly treated with U. S. and other evacuations. The

The Fever is seldom too high, sometimes it is too low for a thorough laudable Eruption. If the Fever is too high, if the patient is plethorick or accustomed to U. S.; take away some Blood but with discretion; if the *Tonsils* are much inflamed with great pain and difficulty in swallowing, use U.S. in the *Jugulars*, Epispasticks ad *Nucham*, encourage the Eruption, or its *succedaneum* a breathing sweat; a profuse *sudor* is equally to be avoided as a continued *Diarrhæa*, either of them confound the distemper in its natural course. In case of colliquations give *ol. Cinamomi, decoct. Alb. Elixir Vitriol, torrified Rhubarb* and the like. As to the specks or sloughs in the *Fauces* (they cast of in course in the benign kind) *Mercurials* inwardly, and the *Gargles* before mentioned topically, are useful; the practice in some Country places of separating them forcibly by *spatulas* is hurtful, because the irritation occasioned thereby induces a further flux upon the part, and the sloughs form again worse conditioned than before. Where the Brain is affected as in *Vigiliæ, jactantia, delirium, Coma, stupor,* &c; glysters, Vesicatories & *suppedanea* are to be used. Where faintness or great prostration of strength, give toasted Bread soaked in some generous Wine and Water, or volatile Spirits in their common drinks; *Bezoars, Testacea* and the like are of no use, the Shop *Cordial Juleps* and mixtures are only sugar'd drams. To enumerate all the other accidental Symptoms which do happen here, in common with other acute diseases, would be trifling.

III. *Consequential ails*, which may be enumerated as in the following articles.

1. *The natural Effects of an intense corrosive scorbutick*

butick like *colliquation of the Blood and Juices*. *Anasarcous* swelling or blotedness of the face, in some to that degree as to shut up the Eyes; the same *Oedemetous* swellings in the extremities; in a few an Infiltration in the *Scrotum;* in some *Petechiæ*, Purple spots, scorbutick like *sugillations* upon the least scratch or bruise; *hæmorrhages* of all sorts, by the Nose, from the Lungs in expectoration, by Stool, by Urine, *Profluviums* in Women *tempore non debito*; these are dismal *phænomina* in the state of any acute Fever, u. g. *Small-Pox*, and scarce any recover; but in our distemper being only short temporary consequential ails, scarce any of them proved mortal, but gave way to a soft milk diet, in some to *Cortex Peruv.* or *Elixir Vitrioli* in others; a Girle æt. 14. with hæmorrhages of several sorts, with Purple spots, and scorbutick like sugillations, recovered, notwithstanding of a very loose *Regimen*. N. B. These were not to be attributed to the *Mercurial* administrations, because they equally happened to those who had taken no Mercury.

2. *Where the defecation has not been compleat*, from want of natural strength, or from catching cold, or from undue evacuations: the *reliquiæ* were thrown off by *Urtications*, by *Vesications* in several parts of the Body, by *serpiginous* eruptions chiefly in the face, by purulent *Pustules*, by Boils, by swellings and *impostumations* in the groin, armpits and other parts of the Body. The most frequent consequential ail of this kind is, when from cold received, the *glands* and cellulary tegument called the *panicula adiposa* in the fore part of the neck becomes infiltrated and obstructed; if not soon resolved by the continued fotus of warm woollens and hot animating applications; the induration increases

creases and spreads every way, so as to suffocate some, in others they sphacelate and become Ulcers mortal or of difficult cure: thus a few have died with us in *Boston*, but many in the Country. By catching cold likeways the *Tonsils* have afterwards inflamed and come to suppuration. In a young Woman the *Tonsils* and *Uvula* being much ulcerated, did unite and coalesce into one mass and remain so; this might have been prevented by frequent gargling.

While these indurations are only in the form of *Kernels* as they are vulgarly called, woollen mufflers, *Empl. de Ranis cum Mercurio* and the like, with gentle *Catharticks*, soon resolves them. *Cataplasms* in this case have done much mischief; because so soon as they are become cold, they act as a chilling damp upon the part, and destroy its vitality. When they arrive to the state of putrid flaccid Ulcerations, digestives and soft fomentations intenerate the part and occasion the Ulcer to spread; spirituous animating desiccative dressings have done better. Exposing the part to the cold, either in state of Tumefaction only, or in the subsequent exulcerations aggravates the ail.

3. *From the violence which the Nerves have suffered in this Illness*; even where the Symptoms were apparently mild, they all complain of great faintness and Universal weakness, particularly in the joints. Some Women have Hysterick affections, in a few upon recovery imbecility of mind or silliness, in some stammering or loss of Speech for a few days, some have had short fits of Melancholy, some were seized with Epileptick fits, but not so as to become habitual. All these disorders soon vanished, as the Patient recovered his Strength in course of time,

and by the help of a restorative cordial *Regimen* and diet.

4. *Other consequential ails in common with other fevers*; particularly where the Strength of nature has been much impared by the distemper it self, or by immoderate evacuations, the Patient is left in a languishing weakness. Where the Eruption has been impeded by being exposed to the cold, or by unseasonable *V. S.* or *Catharticks*; the patient falls into *Hectical wastings*, fatal to some in a very short time. All who underwent immoderate evacuations, were a long time in recovering of their Strength.

SCHOLIA or *some general remarks upon the whole.*
1. *This seems to be a new kind of Epidemical disease.* It is not the same with the *Aphthæ* which have at times prevailed in *Holland*, as described by *Forestus*, and mentioned by *Boerhaave* in his Colleges. *Tournefort* says there is a distemper not uncommon in the *Levant*, viz. a Carbuncle or plague sore in the bottom of the Throat; it carries off children in a few days, but does not affect grown People as does ours. Capt. *Morton* of late *Plymouth* Colony, who wrote many years ago his *New-England Memorial*, says that an. 1650. a disease in the Mouth and Throat prevailed, which proved mortal to many in a short time; but he does not describe it, and mentions nothing of a Fever. In *Boston November* 1719. a slight miliary fever chiefly with children, but was over in two or three days, unless by catching cold it continued appearing and disappearing alternately for some days longer; there was no complaint of the Throat, and no deaths ensued. It is not the same with the sore Throats which are observed from time

time to time in some of our Country Towns, especially in the Winter season: these are Endemial and constitutional, being tumefactious and exulceratious with fluxion in the *Fauces* and Neck; proceeding from an intense scropholous scorbutick, or *Pforick* habit (in such subjects vesications by *Cantharides* did putrifie) without any Eruptive fever: ours have generally an Eruptive fever or tendency that way, so that of those who have died in *Boston*, not above one in seven died of any Throat ail, but of this fever. It is however observable that the Scrophulous and Pforick, are most susceptible of this distemper, and suffer more remarkably.

2. *This Epidemical distemper is no creature of the Seasons*, it having prevailed from *May* 1735. when it first emerged, the whole year or all the Seasons round. *It is no produce of peculiar climates and soils*, because it hath made its appearance in various places from *Pemaquia* in 44 N. Lat. to *Carolina* Southward, and as we are lately informed, it is in our *West India Islands*. It is remarkable that in damp places, as near large Ponds, fresh water Rivers, woodlands, and the like, it has done the greatest execution, as does the *Rot* amongst *Sheep* in fenny Lands.

It is not personally infecting after the rate of the Plague, Small Pox, &c. where every Person is susceptible, excepting a very few *anomolous* constitutions. Children are the most obnoxious to any infection; but with us several Children in the family, where the distemper appeared, have escaped: it is true where it happens in a family, it frequently seizeth severals, as is the case with our Country *Peripneumonick Fevers*, and our Autumnal remitting slow Fevers, which cannot be said to be contagious. The distance in time of Infection to be supposed received from a sick Person, to the time of the distemper's appearing in the supposed infected, could never, with any reasonable allowance of latitude, be reduced to any rule, as in Small-Pox, Measles, &c. We have *Anatomically* inspected Persons who died of it with so intense a *fætor* from the violence of the disease, that some Practioners could not continue in the room; but without being infected our selves or carrying it into families. Many children without reserve, frequent the houses and chambers of the sick, and escape. *It does therefore proceed from some undiscovered quality of the air, affecting only peculiar constitutions of persons and families:* notwithstanding of its being generally favourable, it proves fatal to certain families; many families for this reason have buried all or most of their children, u. g. *Boynton* of *Newbury-Falls* lost his eight children, at *Hampton-Falls* in 5 families died 27 Persons:

3. *This is a very anomalous Illness,* some complain a day or two before they are confined, some are seized as it were instantaneously, it is generally most severe with these last. In some a soreness of the Throat and darting pain there, reaching the Ears, is previous to all other Symptoms; in others the common Symptoms of a fever appear, before any inflamation or specks are perceivable in the *Fauces.* Some have a sore Throat without any perceivable eruption, only a gentle breathing continued Sweat, or an increased insensible perspiration with the peculiar smell of the morbid *effluvia.* Some (but very few) have the cuticular eruptions without any sloughs in the Throat; only the *Tonsils, Uvula, and Velum Palati,* tumified and inflamed; and in a few,

a purulent discharge from some parts deeper than the *Fauces*, that is lower than the sight can reach, these are not without danger. Many of those who died early of a *Necrosis*, had no tumefaction, inflamation or specks in the Throat.

The time of Eruption is very uncertain; in a very few it preceeds the soreness of the Throat, in a few it goes *pari passu* with the affection of the *Fauces*; but generally it is (not much) later than the first complaints of the Throat, in a young Woman it was later by 14 days.

In ruddy complexions the efflorescence is very discernable; it is not so distinctly perceivable in Brunets, Indians, and Negroes; unless the miliary Eruption have a considerable *Relievo* as in some, they generally scale and peal notwithstanding. Sometimes it appears only in the cheeks, sometimes only a few clusters in the extremities. Sometimes the *suffusion* was scarce miliary and vanished insensibly by becoming gradually paler without scaling. Where the Miliary Eruptions were considerable, the extremities peel in scraps or strips like *Exuviæ*; in one or two the nails of the fingers and toes did cast off. The period or continuance of Eruption is sometimes prolonged by weakness of nature, by undue evacuations, or by the Patients being exposed to the cold.

4. In some who were very slightly affected, their Illness was of a much shorter continuance, than is described in the Standard kind. *Most of those who died of the Physician died by immoderate evacuations.* As to the deaths, only a few were occasioned immediately by any distemperature of the Throat; they were generally the effect of the Fever, either by an immediate *Necrosis* at first seizure, or by the
or-

ordinary fatality of Fevers, or by confequential ails. In *Boston* at a medium of the laft eight healthy years (1723. 1724. 1725. 1726 1727. 1728. 1732. and 1733) in the Months of *October, November, December, January, February, March, April* to 18*th May*, died *pr. an.* 268 Whites and Slaves; this year in the fame fpace of time died 382, is 114 *extra* deaths, and may be refonably charged to this Illnefs, it being otherways a healthy time: of thefe 114. about 71 cafes came to my knowledge, whereof in the firft period died 35, in the fecond period 28, and of confequential ails, 8. Of thefe 71, only about 10 can be faid to have died of fore Throats. Of thefe 71 only 9 were upwards of 14 *æt.* According to the neareft eftimate I can make in round numbers, about 1 in 35 have died, that is about 4000 Perfons in *Boston* have had this diftemper, which is about one 4th part of the Inhabitants.

5. The Summer 1735 was unufually wet and chilly with many Eafterly winds, in the Summer & Autumn it prevail'd and was very mortal in feveral Country Towns. In *Boston* it began in Autumn, but did not prevail until Winter, which was not rigid with hard frofts as is ufual, but with a very difagreeable chill in the air, efpecially in the Month of *March* laft, in which Month was our greateft Mortality.

6. *Moft Malignant diftempers affect to throw off their malignancy by fome Emunctory.* The defpumation of this acrid inqination of the juices in our diftemper, that is, its natural *Crifis*, feems to be by the patent and falutary *Emunctories* of the *Fauces* and skin. In corrofive taints, u. g. Venereal and others, a *Mercurial ptyalifm* and fudorifick decoction of the *woods,* anfwer beft; this gave us the hint of promoting
the

the tendency of nature in our Illness, by Mercurials, and gentle breathing Sweats a bed; which with good management seldom fail'd, excepting where the *Necrosis* was irremediable from the beginning.

Some affection of the Throat seems to attend most kinds of Eruptive Fevers. In the *Small-Pox* (even where the pustules and other Symptoms were in the smallest degree) they all complain of a soreness of the Throat, but without ulcerating. In the *Measles* there is a hoarsness, and soreness of the Throat. *In ours* besides the soreness, tumefaction, and inflammation in the *Fauces*; there are specks or sloughs of a mellow white or Cream colour, like those on the inside of the cheeks in a Mercurial ptyalism; the Scrophulous and Venereal ulcers in the Throat are yellow; Aphthæ are more of the nature of *phlyctenæ*; many of our Patients complain of a copperish taste or peppery smart in the Throat, as they express it.

7. *As in all other distempers so in this there do sometimes happen violent Symptoms, meerly from the Regimen and Medicines used;* which on that account are not of that bad consequence, as if they had proceeded from the distemper in its natural course u. g. in some constitutions a *Turbith bolus* operates with violence, so as to occasion shiverings, torsions of the Bowels, and Spasms, as if the Patient were moribund: *Calomel* even in very small doses seizeth the Mouth of some to a very considerable degree of inconveniency.

8 *We did not observe any genuine second seizures.* It is true, being Winter Season, many common sore Throats, that is, relaxations of the *Uvula* and inflammations of the Tonsils; have passed with the less observing practitioners, for the genuine Epedemick

demick and were used accordingly; such have afterwards had this Illness, and was erroneously called a second seizure. N. B. Our *Epidemick* is attended with no cough, unless when complicated with a cold or some old habitual *Tussis:* upon recovery, it leaves frequently a small *catarrhous* colliquation or cough, but of short continuance.

In some after being well, upon catching cold, the *Tonsils* have been inflamed even to suppuration; in others the *Uvula* and *Velum Palati* infiltrated and some *phlyctenæ* or common *Aphthæ*, have appeared. Such have also by some been deem'd as second seizures, and used as such.

After a long continuance of cold chilly Weather, there set in suddenly warm Weather hot as mid Summer. *May* 25th, 26th, *&c.* several children, who formerly had this Eruptive fever, have an efflorescence or *miliary* eruption by the heat, as is not unusual with children in hot weather: this was by mistake of some practitioners and others, called a second seizure.

9. *No conditions of Mankind were exempted* (in our Epidemical Autumnal *dysentery A.* 1734. the Negroes escaped) Europeans, West-India Islanders, Indians and Negroes, of all ages, were equally subject to it: but, as in most Epidemical diseases, it affected Children and the younger Persons more generally.

10. *This is a Real History of the distemper as it appeared in Boston New-England*, taken clinically from the life and not copied. There is no stroak or clause, but what I can vouch by real not imaginary cases. It is founded only upon observations or *phænomina*, that is upon the Symptoms that appeared in the course of this Epidemical disease; it must therefore be of permanent truth.

F I N I S

AN ACCOUNT

Of the Numbers that have died of the

Distemper in the Throat,

Within the Province of

New-Hampshire,

With some Reflections thereon.

July 26. 1736.

by the Revd Jabez Fitch
Minister in Portsmouth.

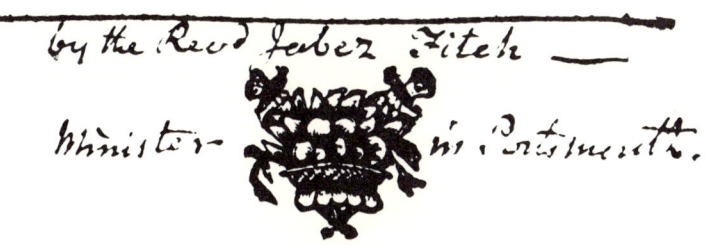

BOSTON:
Printed for *Eleazer Russel* in *Portsmouth.*
1736.

An Account of the Numbers that have died of the *Distemper in the Throat*, within the Province of *New-Hampshire*.

WE in the Province of *New-Hampshire* (with the neighbouring Places) have had frequent Occasion to repeat that doleful Lamentation; *Death is come up into our Windows to cut off the Children from without.* —— And 'tis fit that the extraordinary Mortality which has been among us, should be ever remembered to our Humiliation; in order to which a particular Account of the Numbers that have died, in the several Towns within this Province, mostly the last Winter, is here presented to the Publick.

Tho' some have died of sundry Ages, yet the far greatest part were under *Ten* Years of Age; and Providence having made such a remarkable Distinction, I thought it proper to take Notice of it in the following Account.

In *Portsmouth*,
In the upper part of the Town have died,
Under Ten about ——— — ——— 40.

Between Ten and Fifteen —— —— 6.
Above Twenty —— —— —— 1.

Two have died out of sundry Families, *Four* out of one. Some Families have lost their only Child, and some who had but two Children have lost both of them.

In the lower part of the Town have died,
Under Ten —— —— —— 27.
Between Ten and Twenty —— —— 2.
Above Forty —— —— —— 1.

Two Families lost *three*, one of which lost all, who were buried at the same time. One Family lost *four*.

In that Part of *Portsmouth* call'd the *Plaines*, died,
Under Ten —— —— —— 14.
Between Ten and Twenty —— —— 7.
Above Forty —— —— —— 1.

Two Families lost four a-piece.

In *New Castle* died,
Under Ten —— —— —— 11.

At the *Shoals* have died,
Under Seven —— —— —— 34.
Between Ten and Fifteen —— —— 2.
About Sixty —— —— —— 1.

One Family lost *three*, six Families lost *two* a piece; no Family lost all.

In *Rye* have died,
Under Ten —— —— —— 34.
Between Ten and Fifteen —— —— 6.
Above Fifteen —— —— —— 4.

Two Families lost *three*, one of which lost all, one Family lost *four*, and one *five*.

In *Greenland* have died,

Under Ten ——— ——— ——— 13.
Between Fifteen and Twenty ——— 2.
Between Twenty and Thirty ——— 3.

Two Families lost their only Child.

In *Newington* have died,

Under Ten ——— ——— ——— 16.
Between Ten and Fifteen ——— 4.
Between Fifteen and Twenty ——— 1.

One Family lost *four*, two lost *three*, one of which lost all.

In *Hampton*,

In the first Parish have died,

Under Ten ——— ——— ——— 37.
Between Ten and Fifteen ——— 4.
Between Fifteen and Twenty ——— 4.
Between Twenty and Thirty ——— 8.
Above Thirty ——— ——— ——— 1.
Above *Ninety* ——— ——— ——— 1.

A Woman, who had the manifest Symptoms of the Distemper upon her.

Five Families lost *three* out of each, one Family lost *four*, one lost *five*, within about a Fortnight, the Eldest dying first, and then the next Eldest, 'till the fifth died, and a sixth Child liv'd.

Three Families lost their only Child.

In the second Parish of *Hampton* have died,

Under Ten about ——— ——— 160.
Between Ten and Fifteen about — 25.
Between Fifteen and Twenty ——— 15.
Above Twenty, the eldest of which was nigh Forty ——— ——— ——— 1.

All of these except a small Number died of the late fatal Distemper. Nigh

Nigh Twenty Families loft all their Children, Twenty two loft all their Sons, moft of them being only Sons. One Family loft *seven*, (six Children and a 'Prentice Boy) Two Families loft *six* a piece, Two Families loft *five* a piece, Six Families loft *four* a piece; about fourteen Families loft *three* a piece.

Forty nine died in the Month of *December*.

'Tis suppos'd that more than a sixth part of the Number of Inhabitants in that Parifh have died, within 13 Months.

In *Exeter* have died,

Under Ten	105.
Under Fifteen	13.
Between Fifteen and Twenty	5.
Above Twenty	4.

Two Families loft each *three*, Two Families loft each *four*, Two Families loft each *five*, of which one loft all, and the other had one spar'd.

The Diftemper came into *Exeter* the Beginning of *August*, 1735.

In *Stratham* have died,

Under Ten	18.

One Family loft *four*.

In *Newmarket* have died,

Under Ten	20.
Under Fifteen	1.
Above Thirty	1.

One Family loft *five*, Four Families loft all their Children, one of them *two*, and the other *one* a piece.

In *Kingfton* have died,

Under Ten	96.

Between

Between Ten and Fifteen — — — 10.
Between Fifteen and Twenty — — 5.
Above Twenty — — — — — 1.
Above Thirty — — — — — 1.

One Family that had four Children lost them all, another lost *four* out of *six*; Six Families lost *three* each, one of which had but three.

The Distemper came into *Kingston* the latter end of *May*, 1735.

In *Chester* have died,
Under Ten — — — — — 21.

One Family lost *three*.

In *Dover* have died,
Under Ten — — — 77.
Between Ten and Fifteen — — 5.
Between Fifteen and Twenty — 3.
Between Twenty and Thirty — 3.

Sundry Families lost their only Child, and others that had but *two* lost them both. Five Families lost *three* Children a piece, one of which buried *three* in one Day. Two Families lost *four*, and one of them buried *four* in a Day. One Family lost *six* Children, and *four* were buried at once.

This Distemper began among them in *October*, 1735.

In *Durham* have died,
Under Ten about — — 79.
Under Twenty about — — 15.
Between Twenty and Thirty about — 6.

Three Families lost *four* Children a piece, each of which lost all but one. Three Families lost all. The Distemper began among them in *September*.

In

(6)

In the Lower Parish of *Kittery*, a neighbouring Town to *Portsmouth*, in the other Province have died, —————— —————— —————— —————— 122.

No more than *six* exceeded Fifteen Years, and not more than *six* arriv'd to Fifteen Years. These have died from *June* 1735, to the 16th of *July*, 1736.

According to the foregoing Accounts, there have died,

In *Portsmouth*, ——————————————— 99
In *Newcastle*, ——————————————— 11
At the *Shoals*, ——————————————— 37.
In *Rye*, —————————————————— 44
In *Greenland*, ——————————————— 18.
In *Newington*, ——————————————— 21.
In *Hampton*, ——————————————— 265.
In *Exeter*, including *Newmarket*, ———— 149.
In *Stratham*, ——————————————— 18.
In *Kingston*, ——————————————— 113.
In *Chester*, ——————————————— 21.
In *Dover*, ———————————————— 88.
In *Durham*, ——————————————— 100

The whole Number is, 984

The Distemper began much later in most of the Towns than in the rest.

Since I receiv'd the Account from some of the Towns, the Distemper has come into sundry more Families, and prov'd mortal to some of their Children.

I shall here take Occasion to give some Hints referring to this awful Providence, which every judicious Person may easily enlarge upon in his own Thoughts.

T

The Grave is a Land of Darkness without any Order, which has of late been remarkably seen, in respect of the Age of those that have been brought to it, when so many Younger ones have *gone to their long Home* before the Elder: Yet *every one may be said to die in his own Order*, in respect of God's appointment, who has determin'd the Time of every ones Death, and without whose Providence *not a Sparrow falls to the Ground*; which is a good Reason why we should be silent and submissive under such heavy Trials.

The Death of many Children before they were arriv'd to Years of Discretion, shews the woful Effects of Original Sin, and gives us all just Occasion to make the same humble Reflection on our selves that *David* did, *Behold, I was shapen in Iniquity, and in Sin did my Mother conceive me*: On which Account we might justly have been cut off in the Beginning of our Days, but God has spar'd us in the greatness of his Mercy.

In consideration of the above-mentioned Mortality, which has been chiefly among Children, young ones should be awaken'd to seek after God betimes, when they see those that were as young, or younger than themselves, taken out of the Land of the Living. 'Tis storied of a Child that was noted to be serious and religiously dispos'd, and one asking the Reason hereof, the Child said, I remember I must die; but being told you are likely to live many a Year longer, the Child reply'd, I was lately at a Funeral, where I saw a Grave shorter than my self. Many such sad Spectacles have been to be seen of late. O! that our Children

dren that are arriv'd to any Years of Discretion were so *wise* as to *consider their latter End*, when they have had so frequent Warnings of it. Let Children *remember their Creator* and Redeemer in their early Days, lest these should be all the Days they shall ever have to remember them in. Many dear Children have been laid in their Graves, where *there is no remembrance* of God; those that survive are very inexcusable if they do not lay it to Heart, so as seriously to think of their own dying, and instantly to prepare for it. Let Children consider that they are Sinners, or else they would not be liable to the Stroke of Death, and they have no more assurance of living long, than those Children had, that are now *gone down into Silence*; and let them think sadly what a doleful Condition they will be in, if they should *die in their Sins*; and let them speedily seek an Interest in Jesus Christ, who alone can *save them from their Sins*, and who has said for their Encouragement, *Those that seek me early shall find me*. Let every Child set himself to learn and understand his Catechism, and learn to be *good* betimes. A Pious Child is the Delight of God and Angels. Let every Child learn to pray, and daily go alone and beg of God, that for his Mercy's sake and for Christ's sake, He would forgive his original Sin and all his actual Sins, and that He would *give him a new Heart and put a new Spirit within him*, and cause him to love Him above all, and to take heed of offending Him any more by sinful Thoughts, by wicked Words or vicious Deeds. And O! that all our Children would *remember the Sabbath-Day to keep it holy*, not spending it in Play or Idleness; but in diligent reading of the holy Bible and other good Books, and in a diligent attendance on the Worship of God, Private and Publick. Such Children may hope that God will own them for his Children, that He will take them under his Protection, and that they shall live, so long as an All wise God sees Life would be good for them in this World, and if they should be cut off in their younger Days (as many others have been) God will *satisfy them with long Life, even with Length of Days for ever and ever* in a better World.

It has been observ'd concerning several Children, that their Spirits have been strangely supported in the Agonies of Death; they have shew'd a becoming submission to the Divine Will, and expressed good Hopes of being received to a better World; and utter'd such things as yielded great Consolation to their sorrowful Parents. *Out of the Mouth of Babes and Sucklings* God can *perfect Praise*.

The great Mortality that has been among Children, should make Parents very sensible, that their Children are *uncertain* Comforts, and should quicken them to a faithful Discharge of their Duty towards their Children, by sincerely dedicating them to God, and by training them up in the Knowledge and Fear of God. This will be the way for them to have Comfort in their Children, whether Living or Dying.

Elder ones should adore the Power and Patience of God in prolonging their frail and forfeited Lives; and when they see so many younger and more Innocent than themselves, taken away in such an awful manner, they have reason to *make haste and not delay to keep God's Commandments*, lest He should be provok'd to inflict the like awful Judgment upon them: And some of sundry Ages having been taken away by this woful Diſtemper, it ſhould ſerve for the awakening of all; for what has befallen others may alſo befal any of us.

How awakening eſpecially ſhould the Death of Children be to their Parents? When the firſt-born of the *Egyptians* were ſmitten, they ſaid, *We be all dead Men.* Parents are ſtrangely ſtupid, if the Death of their Children does not put them in mind of their own Mortality. And it ſhould cauſe them to conſider wherein they may have offended God; as the Woman ſaid to the Man of God, *Art thou come to call my Sin to remembrance, and to ſlay my Son?*

But we are not to look upon the immediate ſufferers in this Calamity as greater Sinners than others: Our Saviour checks this cenſorious Humour, *Suppoſe ye that theſe Galileans were Sinners above all the Galileans, becauſe they ſuffer'd ſuch Things? I tell you, nay; but except ye repent, ye ſhall all likewiſe periſh.*

And it muſt be granted, that the Good are often involv'd with the Bad in Publick Calamities; but God can and will make *all things work together for good* to thoſe particular Perſons that *love* his Name.

We read of a hopeful Child in the Houſe of *Jereboam*, that died when he was young, whereby he was taken away from the Evil to come: When hopeful Children are taken away, we know not what Evil may be coming; it concerns us ſpeedily to *acquaint our ſelves with God and make our Peace with Him,* and then Good ſhall come unto us.

Many have been bereav'd of their only Child, and others who have had more Children have been bereav'd of them all; but there is enough in God to make up all our Loſſes in the Creature: And thoſe that ſeek Him in good earneſt ſhall find Him *better to them, than ten Sons.*

Sundry have been raiſed up from a very low eſtate; for *the Lord killeth and maketh alive, He bringeth down*

down to the Grave and bringeth up, which may be understood either of the Distinction He makes between some and others; He *killeth* some, and *maketh* or keepeth others alive, that were attended with the same threatning Symptoms, which must be resolv'd into the Sovereign Pleasure of God; *even so Father, because it seemed good in thine Eyes*; or it may be understood of the Change He makes in the same Person, when He brings down to the Brink of the Grave, and raises up when He pleases. Our Eyes have beheld many such Instances of the Wonder-working Providence of God.

And the Distemper that has prov'd mortal to so many, and very grievous to others, has hitherto been escap'd by many, or they have had it in a moderate Degree. Such distinguishing Favours call for great Thankfulness.

Let those Families whom God has mercifully spar'd, so as not to make any Breach upon them, *not be high-minded, but fear*: The discriminating Goodness of God towards them should *lead them to Repentance,* and they are deeply oblig'd, *If Iniquity be in their Hands, to put it far away, and not to suffer Wickedness to dwell in their Tabernacles.*

Those Parents that have been bereav'd of *one* or *two* of their Children, and have had others spar'd to them, when they consider how many have lost a greater Number, and that several have been bereav'd of all their Children, they have great Reason to be silent both in Heart and Tongue, under the Loss that they have sustained, and to bless the Name of God, that He has not dealt so severely by them, as He has by some others, acknowledging that *it is of the Lord's free and undeserved Mercies that they and their's have not been consumed.*

And it becomes us all *as the Elect of God to put on Bowels of Mercies* towards those sorrowful Parents, that

that have lost sundry of their Children, and especially those that have been bereav'd of all, and we ought to present our fervent Requests before the Throne of Grace in their behalf, that as their *Sorrows abound, so the Divine Consolations may abound* towards them; and tho' they are ready to think as good *Jacob* once did, that *these things are against* them, we should pray that they may be really *for* them, in the Issue, that they may work for their spiritual and everlasting Good.

Tho' Days of Fasting and Prayer have been observ'd in the Beginning of this fatal Calamity, 'tis to be fear'd they were not attended with a suitable Reformation; and therefore God has *answer'd us by terrible things in Righteousness*.

We have for some Years been free from the Calamity of War, but God has many *Arrows* of Judgment in his Quiver, and He can send such Epidemical Diseases among us, as shall be more distressing to the Country in general, than any Wars that we have ever experienced.

We were some Years ago visited with a terrible *Earthquake*, which was a loud Call to Repentance, but the good impressions made by that awful Providence were soon worn off in most Places; tis no wonder then that God proceeds to real inflictions of Judgments, when we have forgotten the awful Warning He has given us thereof.

The Progress of the late Distemper has been very strange in its passing from one Town to another, after a considerable space of Time, and in its long remaining in one part of a Town, before it has pass'd into other parts, and in its returning where it seem'd to be quite gone and the Fears of it were blown over; on these Accounts the Act of Providence is the more visible in sending it, and we are led to look beyond natural Causes to the Hand of God, to whom we are

We chiefly concern'd to apply our selves, for the Removal of this awful Calamity.

We know not what the Designs of Providence may be, but by what we hear of the spreading of this Distemper in other parts of the Country, it seems as if the Lord *were risen up out of his holy Habitation* and coming forth in this awful manner against the whole Continent. It therefore concerns all Places and Persons to *prepare to meet the Lord* in the way of his Judgments, by unfeigned Repentance and humble Supplication, that He may *turn from the fierceness of his Anger*.

The Loss of so many Children, whom if it had pleas'd God that they had liv'd, might have built up many Families, will be a great Prevention of the Growth and Increase of the Country; and ought therefore to be lookt upon as a Frown of Providence upon the Land in general, as well as a sore Affliction to the Parents in particular.

We should seriously enquire *wherefore* the Almighty has thus *contended* with us? We have Reason to look upon the *strange* unusual Distemper that has prevail'd among us, as the Fruit of *strange* Sins. Have not many *strangely* neglected the great Salvation? Have not many Professors of Religion *strangely* contradicted their Profession in their Lives? Have not many been *strangely* guilty of prophaning God's sacred Name and Sabbaths? Have not many People been *strangely* addicted some to one Vice and some to another? To Pride, Envy, Malice, Evil speaking, Fraud and Injustice, Strife and Contention, Sensuality & Intemperance, or to a worldly Spirit, whereby they have been dispos'd to be *strangely* grasping after the World for the sake of their Children: But God by the late awful Providence, has shew'd how vain a thing it is for Parents to be inordinate in their Desires and Endeavours, to lay up for their

Chil-

Children, when they know not whether their Children shall live to enjoy what they have laid up for them.

It concerns us all to *search and try our Ways, and turn unto the Lord*, and *diligently hearken to his Voice*, the Voice of his Rod as well as Word, *and to do that which is right in his Sight, and to give ear to his Commandments and keep all his Statutes*; we may then expect the like Favour from Him, which He promis'd to his ancient People; *I will put none of those Diseases upon thee, which I have brought upon the Egyptians; for I am the Lord that healeth thee.*

F I N I S.

Medicine & Society
In America

An Arno Press/New York Times Collection

Alcott, William A. **The Physiology of Marriage.** 1866. New Introduction by Charles E. Rosenberg.

Beard, George M. **American Nervousness: Its Causes and Consequences.** 1881. New Introduction by Charles E. Rosenberg.

Beard, George M. **Sexual Neurasthenia.** 5th edition. 1898.

Beecher, Catharine E. **Letters to the People on Health and Happiness.** 1855.

Blackwell, Elizabeth. **Essays in Medical Sociology.** 1902. Two volumes in one.

Blanton, Wyndham B. **Medicine in Virginia in the Seventeenth Century.** 1930.

Bowditch, Henry I. **Public Hygiene in America.** 1877.

Bowditch, N[athaniel] I. **A History of the Massachusetts General Hospital: To August 5, 1851.** 2nd edition. 1872.

Brill, A. A. **Psychanalysis: Its Theories and Practical Application.** 1913.

Cabot, Richard C. **Social Work: Essays on the Meeting-Ground of Doctor and Social Worker.** 1919.

Cathell, D. W. **The Physician Himself and What He Should Add to His Scientific Acquirements.** 2nd edition. 1882. New Introduction by Charles E. Rosenberg.

The Cholera Bulletin. Conducted by an Association of Physicians. Vol. I: Nos. 1–24. 1832. All published. New Introduction by Charles E. Rosenberg.

Clarke, Edward H. **Sex in Education; or, A Fair Chance for the Girls.** 1873.

Committee on the Costs of Medical Care. **Medical Care for the American People:** The Final Report of The Committee on the Costs of Medical Care, No. 28. [1932].

Currie, William. **An Historical Account of the Climates and Diseases of the United States of America.** 1792.

Davenport, Charles Benedict. **Heredity in Relation to Eugenics.** 1911. New Introduction by Charles E. Rosenberg.

Davis, Michael M. **Paying Your Sickness Bills.** 1931.

Disease and Society in Provincial Massachusetts: Collected Accounts, 1736–1939. 1972.

Earle, Pliny. **The Curability of Insanity: A Series of Studies.** 1887.

Falk, I. S., C. Rufus Rorem, and Martha D. Ring. **The Costs of Medical Care:** A Summary of Investigations on The Economic Aspects of the Prevention and Care of Illness, No. 27. 1933.

Faust, Bernhard C. **Catechism of Health:** For the Use of Schools, and for Domestic Instruction. 1794.

Flexner, Abraham. **Medical Education in the United States and Canada:** A Report to The Carnegie Foundation for the Advancement of Teaching, Bulletin Number Four. 1910.

Gross, Samuel D. **Autobiography of Samuel D. Gross, M.D.,** with Sketches of His Contemporaries. Two volumes. 1887.

Hooker, Worthington. **Physician and Patient; or, A Practical View of the Mutual Duties, Relations and Interests of the Medical Profession and the Community.** 1849.

Howe, S. G. **On the Causes of Idiocy.** 1858.

Jackson, James. **A Memoir of James Jackson, Jr., M.D.** 1835.

Jennings, Samuel K. **The Married Lady's Companion, or Poor Man's Friend.** 2nd edition. 1808.

The Maternal Physician; a Treatise on the Nurture and Management of Infants, from the Birth until Two Years Old. 2nd edition. 1818. New Introduction by Charles E. Rosenberg.

Mathews, Joseph McDowell. **How to Succeed in the Practice of Medicine.** 1905.

McCready, Benjamin W. **On the Influences of Trades, Professions, and Occupations in the United States, in the Production of Disease.** 1943.

Mitchell, S. Weir. **Doctor and Patient.** 1888.

Nichols, T[homas] L. **Esoteric Anthropology: The Mysteries of Man.** [1853].

Origins of Public Health in America: Selected Essays, 1820–1855. 1972.

Osler, Sir William. **The Evolution of Modern Medicine.** 1922.

The Physician and Child-Rearing: Two Guides, 1809–1894. 1972.

Rosen, George. **The Specialization of Medicine:** with Particular Reference to Ophthalmology. 1944.

Royce, Samuel. **Deterioration and Race Education.** 1878.

Rush, Benjamin. **Medical Inquiries and Observations.** Four volumes in two. 4th edition. 1815.

Shattuck, Lemuel, Nathaniel P. Banks, Jr., and Jehiel Abbott. **Report of a General Plan for the Promotion of Public and Personal Health.** Massachusetts Sanitary Commission. 1850.

Smith, Stephen. **Doctor in Medicine** and Other Papers on Professional Subjects. 1872.

Still, Andrew T. **Autobiography of Andrew T. Still,** with a History of the Discovery and Development of the Science of Osteopathy. 1897.

Storer, Horatio Robinson. **The Causation, Course, and Treatment of Reflex Insanity in Women.** 1871.

Sydenstricker, Edgar. **Health and Environment.** 1933.

Thomson, Samuel. **A Narrative, of the Life and Medical Discoveries of Samuel Thomson.** 1822.

Ticknor, Caleb. **The Philosophy of Living; or, The Way to Enjoy Life and Its Comforts.** 1836.

U.S. Sanitary Commission. **The Sanitary Commission of the United States Army:** A Succinct Narrative of Its Works and Purposes. 1864.

White, William A. **The Principles of Mental Hygiene.** 1917.